THE SOCIOLOGY OF
HIV TRANSMISSION

THE SOCIOLOGY OF HIV TRANSMISSION

Michael Bloor

SAGE Publications
London • Thousand Oaks • New Delhi

© Michael Bloor 1995

First published 1995

All rights reserved. No part of this publication may be
reproduced, stored in a retrieval system, transmitted or utilized
in any form or by any means, electronic, mechanical,
photocopying, recording or otherwise, without permission in
writing from the Publishers.

 SAGE Publications Ltd
6 Bonhill Street
London EC2A 4PU

SAGE Publications Inc
2455 Teller Road
Thousand Oaks, California 91320

SAGE Publications India Pvt Ltd
32, M-Block Market
Greater Kailash – I
New Delhi 110 048

British Library Cataloguing in Publication data

A catalogue record for this book is
available from the British Library

ISBN 0-8039-8749 8
ISBN 0-8039-8750 1 (pbk)

Library of Congress catalog card number 95-068522

Typeset by M Rules
Printed in Great Britain by Biddles Ltd, Guildford

Contents

To Chris and Alice

List of Tables

Acknowledgements

In the writing of this book I have incurred many debts which I am glad to have this opportunity to acknowledge. Sally Macintyre, Director of the Medical Research Council's Medical Sociology Unit in Glasgow, first suggested that I write this book. At that time I had responsibility, under Sally's direction, for a series of studies on HIV/AIDS (funded by MRC, ESRC and WHO) being conducted within the unit and collaboratively with other researchers based elsewhere in Glasgow. I owe a debt to Sally and also to all those others with whom I worked and collaborated on HIV/AIDS research in Glasgow – Marina Barnard, Pete Beharrell, Andrew Boddy, Rob Covell, Sarah Cunningham Burley, John Eldridge, Andrew Finlay, Martin Frischer, David Goldberg, Gill Green, Steve Green, Sally Haw, Jenny Kitzinger, Neil McKeganey, David Miller, Steve Platt, Greg Philo, Avril Taylor, Danny Wight and Kevin Williams. I owe a special debt to Marina Barnard, Andrew Finlay and Neil McKeganey, each of whom on different occasions acted as my co-fieldworker in the collection of the data on male prostitution reported in Chapter 5. That work was supported by the Medical Research Council; Greater Glasgow Health Board supplied the free condoms that we distributed (my thanks here to Elizabeth Wilson and Susan Carr). This book has a broader scope than the reporting of those Glasgow studies, but much of the thinking that lies behind the writing was begun at that time and in the context of that work.

When I left Glasgow to come to Cardiff I had only succeeded in drafting a couple of the chapters which follow. I was therefore fortunate that Paul Atkinson, Head of the School of Social and Administrative Studies, was as keen as I was that the book should be completed: I am grateful for his support. Others in Cardiff have also been helpful with references, ideas and support. I would particularly like to thank Sara Delamont, Marian Garside, Mart Read, Clive Rees and Heather Snidle. Various colleagues in Britain and abroad have been helpful in discussions and in the loan of unpublished material. I should particularly thank Gary Albrecht, Marina Barnard, Isobel Bowler, Peter Davies, Martin Frischer, Graham Hart, Jeff Kelly, Jenny Kitzinger, Tim Rhodes, Gerry Stimson, Peter Weatherburn and Danny Wight. David Goldberg kindly checked the overview of clinical aspects of HIV in the introductory chapter.

Some of the material here has also been reported in rather different forms elsewhere. I am grateful to the editors of *AIDS Care* and to Carfax Publishing Company for permission to reprint material from M. Bloor, N. McKeganey, A. Finlay and M. Barnard (1992) 'The inappropriateness of psychosocial models of risk behaviour for understanding HIV-related risk practices among Glasgow male prostitutes', *AIDS Care*, 4: 131-137. I am grateful to the editor of *Medical Anthropology Quarterly* and the American Anthropological Association for permission to reprint material from M. Bloor, M. Barnard, A. Finlay and N. McKeganey (1993) 'HIV-related risk practices among Glasgow male prostitutes: reframing concepts of risk behavior', *Medical Anthropology Quarterly*, 7: 152–169. I am grateful to the Editorial Board and Blackwell Publishers for permission to reprint material from M. Bloor, M. Frischer and A. Taylor et al. (1994) 'Tideline and turn? Possible reasons for the continuing low prevalence among injecting drug users in Glasgow', *Sociological Review*, 42: 738–757. I am grateful to the editors of *Sociology of Health and Illness* and to Blackwell Publishers for permission to reprint material that originally appeared in M. Bloor (1995) 'A user's guide to contrasting theories of HIV-related risk behaviour', in Volume 17, issue 4 of *Sociology of Health and Illness*, a special monograph on *The Sociology of Risk* edited by John Gabe, to be published in July 1995. I am grateful to David Fitzsimmons and his co-editors, the National AIDS Trust and to Cassell for permission to reprint material from M. Bloor (1995) 'HIV-related risk behaviour among international travellers: an overview', in D. Fitzsimmons et al. (eds) *The Economic and Social Impact of AIDS in Europe*, London: Cassell. Some of the material in Chapter 6 is reworked from a background paper I wrote for the Health Education Authority and a technical paper I wrote for the Welsh Health Planning Forum.

Publishing projects have a tendency to linger on past deadlines. At least, this one did. I am grateful first to Karen Phillips and then to Krysia Domaszewicz at Sage for their patience and good advice. There was a dreary period when the only opportunity that I had to grind on with this book was to get up ridiculously early on Sunday mornings. For that reason not least, my family deserve this book's dedication.

Abbreviations

AIDS	acquired immune deficiency syndrome
ARC	AIDS related complex
AZT	zidovudine
CDC	Centers for Disease Control
CMV	cytomegalovirus
DMD	Duchenne muscular dystrophy
EBV	Epstein–Barr virus
EU	European Union
GUM	genito-urinary medicine
HBM	'health beliefs' model
HIV	human immunodeficiency virus
IDU	injecting drug user
KS	Kaposi's sarcoma
MACS	Multicenter AIDS Cohort Study (USA)
MESMAC	Men who have Sex with Men – Action in the Community (project)
NATSSAL	National Survey of Sexual Attitudes and Lifestyles
PCP	pneumocystis carinii pneumonia
PWA	person with AIDS
STD	sexually transmitted disease
TB	tuberculosis
WRAP	Women, Risk and AIDS Project

1

Introduction

Like most researchers involved in the HIV/AIDS epidemic, I find that it is individuals who stand sharpest in my memory. Two cases out of many will suffice for illustration (I have changed some of the background circumstances for obvious reasons). On one occasion, I and a fellow researcher were chatting one afternoon to a young man outside a public lavatory as part of an ethnographic study of male prostitution and HIV-related risk behaviour. He was explaining that he never worked at the prostitution sites in the evenings, preferring to spend the evenings in cosy domesticity with his girlfriend and child. He falsely told his girlfriend that he simply ripped off 'punters' (prostitutes' clients) encountered at the lavatories, rather than performing any sexual services. I asked if he and his girlfriend used condoms: he shyly confided that there was no current necessity as she was expecting another baby.

Again, I recall interviewing an injecting drug user at a needle exchange as part of preliminary work in the development of a standardised interview schedule for use by the World Health Organisation. I asked him to tell me about the last occasion on which he had shared his 'works' (injecting equipment): he looked embarrassed, dropped his voice although we were alone in the room, and then hesitatingly confided that it had happened in a well-known residential drug treatment/detox facility.

To me, these stories have a poignant and tragic character (although I imagine that some readers may react to them with outrage at what they perceive to be multiple betrayals of trust). But they stand stark in my memory for the lessons they teach rather than the feelings they evoke: all narratives have instrumental functions. The above narratives could emphasise several points (for example, the rigid compartmentalisation some prostitutes establish between their private and commercial sexual relationships), but in my mind the first story best illustrates the strange asymmetry with which we are all afflicted through health education messages which emphasise our vulnerability to infection from others, but not our propensity to unknowingly infect others: to my respondent, condoms only had a contraceptive function in his domestic life; accustomed to thinking of HIV as an infection he could catch from others, he did not think of it at all as a disease he could pass on to his family. The second case illustrates a point which, at the time of the encounter (late 1980s), struck me with the force of novelty, namely that residential drug treatment units could unwittingly serve the same role in the epidemic as prisons, in mixing together drug injectors from different localities without access to clean injecting equipment.

Of course, most of the narratives which circulate concerning the epidemic are mythic in character – contemporary urban myths of the same order as those which tell of the unauthorised removal of a drugged teenager's kidney, after a kidnapping from a rave club. A widely popular HIV/AIDS myth which occurs in several related forms is the morning-after message from the 'revenge' infector. Sometimes it is a message written in lipstick or shaving foam in the bathroom by the already departed bedfellow. Other times, it is a message opened on the return flight from the romantic holiday. But the content of the message is always the same: 'Welcome to the AIDS Club.' This is in fact a new version of a very old song: Daniel Defoe's account of the Great Plague in seventeenth-century London (Defoe, 1986) critically appraises stories of 'revenge infection' purportedly perpetrated by refugees from the pestilence on householders in areas outside London.

Urban myths address topics of contemporary concern and unease. They often have an overt or underlying sexual theme, they stress the innocent and unprotected character of the victims in the narrative, they often refer to recent cultural and institutional change, and they often serve to legitimise demands for surveillance and control. They have been analysed in these terms by sociologists: the classic analysis of a contemporary myth is that undertaken by Morin (1971) concerning a story that swept the French provincial city of Orleans and that claimed that local schoolgirls were being kidnapped from the changing rooms of (Jewish-owned) boutiques and being sold to white slavers; more recently, Dingwall (1993) has studied the rave club kidnapping-and-kidney-removal story that circulated in the East Midlands of England.

The suitability of the HIV/AIDS epidemic as a topic for urban myth-making hardly needs stating – the marginalised and vilified character of many persons with AIDS (drug injectors, gay men, black Africans), the popular dichotomy (most evident in vampire stories) which divides sexual partners into guilty predators and innocent victims, and so on. The thematic contents of urban myths of the epidemic are echoed in much media coverage of the epidemic (Beharrell, 1992; Kitzinger and Miller, 1992). Yet the mythology is as far from scientific understanding of the epidemic as the Dracula story is from scientific zoology.

This book aims to contest those myths by providing an overview or summary statement of our very considerable contemporary knowledge of the sociology of HIV transmission. The scientific gains have been, by any yardstick, great, but their penetration into the public consciousness has been very limited. The 'revenge infection' myth is a case in point. The 'Welcome to the AIDS Club' story has a very wide circulation. The myth has been amplified by popular news stories such as that surrounding the allegations in the UK that a Birmingham haemophiliac had knowingly infected a number of his heterosexual partners. Possibly the best known popular book on the epidemic, Shilts's *And the Band Played On* (1987) fosters the same myth with its account of the large role allegedly played in the early days of the American epidemic by a deceased Air Canada steward, the so-called 'Patient Zero'. In contrast, the research evidence indicates that those who know themselves to be infected are more likely to reduce their risk behaviour than increase it (see, for example, Kelly et al.'s [1989] study of gay men, or McKeganey's [1990] study of injecting drug users). Of course, one's HIV status is frequently unknown and, like the male prostitute with his girlfriend, the possibility that one may be unwittingly transmitting the virus to one's partner may go entirely unconsidered. But the negative evidence on 'revenge infection' is hardly known outside of small academic and specialist circles: so strong is the grip of the 'revenge infection' myth on public consciousness that, in almost every non-specialist audience I have ever encountered, I have found that the unexamined assumption predominates that HIV infection is knowingly transmitted by many persons with HIV/AIDS.

The non-specialist reader will find here a number of other pieces of social science evidence on the epidemic that accord ill with popular and media images of the epidemic. There is the evidence, for example, that it is the safer sexual practices of those maligned and victimised 'Typhoid Marys', female prostitutes, which have been the main bulwark against a rapid, African-style, heterosexual HIV epidemic in the developed world. Further, the dramatic change in the sexual behaviour of men who have sex with men pre-dated the large-scale government health education campaigns and can be ascribed instead to self-help initiatives and major cultural changes within the gay community. And again, IDUs (injecting drug users) have repeatedly been characterised as irresponsible, driven solely by the need to service their addictions, impervious and unresponsive to public health messages; yet the drug-injecting populations of the developed world have now achieved, like men who have sex with men, a major reduction in risk behaviour.

It is not only among non-specialist audiences that this scientific effort by sociologists (*and* anthropologists, epidemiologists, statisticians and psychologists) has gone unremarked. Even among their peers, this large-scale research effort is almost unnoticed. Few of the main research findings have been published in the major British sociological journals (although they have found homes elsewhere). Many sociologists are largely unaware of the part their colleagues have played in the inter-disciplinary teams that have conducted some of the largest and most ambitious social research projects ever undertaken, such as the National Survey of Sexual Attitudes and Lifestyles (NATSSAL) – the first ever national UK survey of sexual behaviour, based on a random sample of 19,000 households (Wellings et al., 1994). Much work remains to be done, but much has also been achieved. It is my hope that this book will increase the recognition of that collective achievement.

To attempt an overview of the social transmission of HIV may seem to some to be a hopeless task. I have had to limit my aims with care. The book does not include sociological studies of the treatment and illness experience of HIV-positive persons and those living with AIDS: it is concerned solely with risk behaviour. It aims to be synoptic rather than comprehensive. A comprehensive treatment is impossible: any reader who thinks otherwise is advised to visit just one of the great international AIDS conferences and discover there literally thousands of scientific presentations. And although, in the judgement of many, the pace of sociological research in this area has begun to slow down, any attempt at a comprehensive treatment would very quickly be rendered obsolete. That a synoptic treatment is needed is something I have become well aware of in the course of teaching both sociology and medical students and addressing various and diverse audiences on social transmission. Inevitably, the content of the book is coloured by my experience as a researcher within Britain. But this is a global epidemic and I have tried to redress any tendency to dwell exclusively on British work, not least in devoting separate chapters and chapter sections to the developing world epidemic. Even a synoptic treatment is a daunting goal.

The plan of the book is straightforward but also rough and ready. The next two chapters are concerned largely with the social epidemiology of the HIV epidemic in its different manifestations in the developing world and in the developed world, but within both chapters I have allowed myself occasional digressions into more explicitly sociological and anthropological territory where there was a narrative justification. In these social epidemiology chapters it is accepted that different patterns of HIV prevalence may be partly understood as a consequence of local differences in the time-period of the epidemic and as a consequence of biological factors, most notably the differential distribution of co-factors such as chancroid (a sexually transmitted disease which results in bloody genital sores) that serve to amplify the transmissibility of HIV. But it is argued that the different patterns of HIV prevalence are fundamentally shaped by differences in risk behaviour.

The brief chapters on social epidemiology are followed, in Chapter 4, by reports of sociological studies of risk behaviour. This allows a critical overview of some of the previous epidemiological thinking. The 'core groups hypothesis' is examined, the favoured epidemiological explanation for the much more rapid heterosexual HIV epidemic found in sub-Saharan Africa and some Asian countries, an explanation which allocates a central role to prostitution practice. Parallels are drawn between studies of risk practices in different social contexts (among men who have sex with men, among injecting drug users, in private and commercial heterosexual encounters) which stress the important role played by types of relationship (sexual relationships and syringe-sharing relationships) and other situational factors in understanding differences in risk behaviour: risk behaviour is seen to be associated with intimacy and trust, or with strategic power relations.

The research findings reported in Chapter 4 are then, in Chapter 5, related to the different theoretical models of risk behaviour current in the sociological literature. The particular case of unsafe commercial sexual behaviour among male prostitutes is used as an exemplar of some of the main difficulties with current theories. The bones of a phenomenological approach are used as a heuristic basis for alternative theorising.

The conclusion attempts a summary of the foregoing and draws the reader's attention, not just to the variable content of our current sociological knowledge of the epidemic, but also to the varying certitude of that knowledge – to some of the problems of interpretation and to some of the research tasks that remain. Finally, the book takes up the easy criticism of an anonymous publisher's reader: 'theories of themselves may be interesting to some sociologists but to many of those working in the field it is the practical consequences of such [*sic*] that are the greatest concern'. Rather than dismiss this as yet another attack on the Ivory Tower (an attack I would feel quite comfortable about, having spent hundreds of hours handing out free condoms and advice/information packs), I seek to finish the manuscript with a consideration of the implications for disease prevention of the earlier theoretical discussion. There is nothing so practical as a good theory.

The remainder of this introduction provides a brief overview of clinical aspects of the disease for non-specialist readers. More detailed accounts are available in clinical texts (for example, Houweling and Coutinho, 1991a).

HIV, Human Immunodeficiency Virus, is a retrovirus. Retroviruses are widespread among animals; some are relatively harmless, some are cancer-producing and some are of the lentivirinae family – 'slow' viruses leading to long-term degenerative diseases. Prior to the isolation of the HIV-1 retrovirus in 1983 (by a group at the Institut Pasteur in Paris), only two human retroviruses had been identified – HTLV-I and HTLV-II, both associated with leukaemia. In 1986, a new type of HIV

(HIV-2) was isolated from West African AIDS patients who were not infected with HIV-1. Both viruses, like influenza viruses, are characterised by considerable variation in local strains; this variability in virus strains poses a problem for vaccine development.

A few weeks after infection a minority of those infected will experience and present a transitory flu-like illness, with variable signs and symptoms. The body develops antibodies to the virus and a period of dormancy sets in. Tests of HIV positivity are based on tests for the antibody (this is why those who fear a recent infection and go for tests must return for a second test three months after their most recent risk activity has occurred – to allow time for the antibodies to develop). The period of dormancy is misnamed in that, far from a period of inactivity occurring, the constantly replicating virus is engaged in a long-running struggle with the body's immune defences (Ho et al., 1995).

The length of the period of dormancy varies greatly (some HIV-infected persons have remained AIDS-free for fourteen years or more: Buchbinder et al., 1994), but typically several years after infection the body's immune system begins to function progressively less effectively. This occurs through a depletion and impairment of the T4 cells, a type of white blood cell. With a much-reduced T4 cell count, the infected person is prey to the kinds of life-threatening infections and tumours that patients suffer following prolonged immunosuppressive therapy (as in cancer patients treated by prolonged chemotherapy). HIV-infected patients with such disorders are defined as having AIDS, the Acquired Immune Deficiency Syndrome. Two of the most commonly found AIDS-related disorders are pneumocystis carinii pneumonia ('PCP') and the skin cancer, Kaposi's sarcoma ('KS'). It was the upsurge in demand in 1981 for the drug pentamidine, used to treat PCP, that alerted the US Centers for Disease Control to the possibility of an epidemic. In the developing world AIDS sufferers frequently show severe diarrhoea and weight-loss – the 'Slim Disease'. In Africa, AIDS and tuberculosis (TB) often co-exist; there is a possible association with AIDS increasing the patient's susceptibility to TB and TB increasing the patient's susceptibility to HIV infection and vulnerability to AIDS-related illnesses.

Improved treatments have been developed for the opportunistic infections that plague AIDS sufferers and for diseases such as Kaposi's sarcoma, but at the time of writing the only proven treatments that inhibit viral replication are zidovudine (AZT), which sometimes produces side-effects such as anaemia, and the drugs DDI and DDC, both singly and in combination. There is no proven therapy which can eliminate the virus, and disappointing results have come from trials of AZT treatment for asymptomatic HIV-positive patients, trials set in train to discover whether progression to AIDS is slowed by such treatment. Vaccine development is slow, not only because of factors such as HIV mutation and divergent HIV strains, but also because of difficulties in conducting trials of candidate vaccines – for example, the long dormancy period suggests that trials will have to be conducted over a considerable time-period. For the foreseeable future, prevention remains the only effective way of combating the epidemic. And it may always remain the most cost-effective option.

The main HIV transmission routes are widely understood – unprotected vaginal and anal intercourse, the sharing of contaminated needles and syringes, and mother-to-child transmission. Transmission formerly occurred via blood transfusion, blood products (such as Factor VIII for haemophilia A), donated semen, organs and tissues; the risk of such transmission is now extremely small, following the development of screening, testing, heat-inactivation and other procedures. Transmission is also possible via unprotected oro-genital sex, particularly in association with oral ulcers or bleeding gums, but the risk is less than in unprotected vaginal and anal intercourse.

HIV has been isolated from saliva in infected persons, but rarely and with low efficiency; moreover the virus rapidly becomes inactive in saliva. The risk of such transmission is extremely remote and of no epidemiological importance. Early speculation that transmission could occur via insect bites (and particularly through mosquito bites) has proved unfounded.

Transmissibility varies between the different transmission routes. From studies in the developed world, it appears that transmissibility is greater in unprotected anal sex than in unprotected vaginal sex and in the latter case is greater from men to women than from women to men. There are different methods of needle-sharing and these too carry different risks of infection. Transmissibility also certainly varies according to the different infectiousness and probably varies according to the different susceptibility of individuals. Infectiousness is thought to be greatest when an individual is in the earliest and later stages of HIV Disease – before antibodies have developed and after progression to AIDS has occurred. Once antibodies have developed, and while the infected person remains well, infection can still occur but that individual's infectiousness is thought to be reduced. Transmissibility is amplified by the presence of 'co-factors'. Other sexually transmitted diseases (STDs) may be important co-factors, particularly those which produce genital lesions and ulceration (for example, chancroid).

The variable transmissibility of HIV from mother to child is thought to be patterned in a similar way to the above, with the infection risk greatest among children born to infected women who have progressed to AIDS. Data from a European collaborative study of perinatal HIV transmission indicates a transmission rate from mother to child of between 12 and 17 per cent (Peckham, 1993); this is a lower rate than that found in African studies. AZT treatment administered to the mother during pregnancy appears to reduce transmission rates. Infection occurs both within the uterus and particularly intra-partum (that is, during delivery). Breast-feeding is another possible medium of infection, with breast-fed children of HIV-positive mothers twice as likely to be infected as bottle-fed children; the infection risk is greatest among children born to women who only became infected after they had given birth (before the development of antibodies). However, the World Health Organisation is advising the continuation of breast-feeding in developing countries because of the risk to bottle-fed children of other infections due to contaminated water supplies and because of the loss of the protection afforded by the mother's milk.

Latex condoms are an effective barrier, not just against HIV but also against other STDs. Strengthened condoms are necessary for anal sex if tearing is not to occur, but even strengthened condoms in anal sex have a higher failure rate than that of most non-strengthened condoms in vaginal sex. Some condoms are treated with spermicides which have been shown to inactivate HIV, but at least one commonly used spermicide is thought to sometimes produce an adverse reaction, possibly leading to the genital ulceration of the receptive partner. Increasing drug injectors' access to unused injecting equipment has been the most widespread successful means of reducing syringe-sharing. In many American states where syringe-exchanges are illegal small containers of bleach have been distributed to facilitate sterilisation of existing injecting equipment. A similar practice has been introduced into Scottish prisons, where sterilisation tablets have been distributed.

No overview of the epidemic can ignore the persistent and well-publicised criticisms that have been voiced, questioning the scientific link between the virus and the syndrome. Some of these criticisms have come from within academe (for example, Duisberg, 1993), but it is from sections of the press that these criticisms have come loudest and longest, with the UK's *Sunday Times* science correspondent, Neville Hodgkinson, the most prominent of all (see, for example, 'Conspiracy of silence' in the *Sunday Times* of 3 April 1994). The criticisms are multiple and various – that there is no African epidemic, that AIDS victims are dying of the effects of toxic treatments or of recreational drugs – but they centre on the nature of the epidemiological link between HIV and AIDS.

Critics claim that the HIV/AIDS epidemiological link is spurious, that there are AIDS cases without HIV infection and HIV infection cases without AIDS. The latter is to be expected, given the long period between infection and AIDS progression that was described earlier, but longitudinal studies of cohorts of HIV-positive individuals show year-by-year increases in the cumulative totals of those individuals developing AIDS. It is too early to say whether infection with this lentivirus will result in progression to AIDS in *all* cases: there are of course many other human diseases where a proportion of those infected remain asymptomatic carriers. However, the experience with animal lentiviruses does not give grounds for optimism.

Of much more potential seriousness is the claim that AIDS may often develop without prior HIV infection. If this were the case, then the epidemiological link would indeed be highly suspect. As was stated earlier, immune deficiency can occur in a number of ways, most notably as a consequence of cancer treatment. However, cases are extremely rare of HIV-negative patients with moderate to severe immune deficiency that are not attributable to a known specific cause such as immunosuppressive therapy: at a specially convened session on this topic at the VIII International AIDS Conference in Amsterdam in 1992, James Curran, director of HIV/AIDS at the American public health monitoring body in Atlanta – the Centers for Disease Control – stated that the Centers had received reports of only six such cases in recent years. The causal epidemiological link between HIV and AIDS appears to be securely founded. This text is written in the belief that AIDS can be prevented by the prior prevention of HIV infection.

2

The Epidemic of HIV Infection in the Developing World

The same set of statistics on unemployment trends may be used by one politician to claim failure for the government's policies (a continued rise in unemployment) and by a second politician to claim success for the same policies (unemployment is now increasing much less rapidly than in previous months – the recession is over). Disraeli's sardonic juxtaposition ('lies, damn' lies and statistics') notwithstanding, statistics have a privileged status in Western culture. As a mode of representation of social reality, statistics alone may claim the status of scientific 'facts'; their self-evident 'objective' status establishes their superiority over alternative models of discourse such as journalists' reportage or personal anecdote. It is this very superiority, this privileged status, that attracts Disraelian contumely and popular distrust, since statistics may be used to proclaim the objective and scientific truth of a contested point of view. Statistics on epidemic spread are a mode of representation no different in character to the unemployment statistics; they are discursive practices used variously to promote homophobia or xenophobia in the name of social hygiene, to advance the sectional claims of occupational groups (counsellors, drugs outreach workers, health educators, social researchers), and to argue for changes in resource allocation.

Data on current rates of infection and, more importantly, projections of future epidemic spread, are inevitably controversial. When James Chin, the World Health Organisation's chief AIDS epidemiologist, stood up to give his keynote speech at the 1991 international AIDS conference in Florence he faced an audience of Disraelian sceptics. Making the usual epidemiological distinction between rates of incidence (new cases, usually new cases per annum) and rates of prevalence (the cumulative total of infected cases in the population), Dr Chin suggested that, in the developed world, HIV had spread most rapidly in the 1980s. In most Western countries the incidence of HIV peaked in the mid-1980s. Because of the long dormancy period before the onset of AIDS, this decline in HIV incidence in the West has not yet been followed by a decline in AIDS incidence. But Chin expected annual AIDS cases in the developed countries to peak before the mid-1990s (Chin, 1991).

To some in his audience, Dr Chin was being too sanguine about the course of the epidemic in the West. One need not have a professional axe to grind to be concerned about, say, the possibility of a long-term but slow-building epidemic of heterosexually transmitted HIV (see Phyllida Brown's account of reactions to Chin's address – Brown, 1991). And projections for England and Wales in the revised Day Report (PHLS Working Group, 1993), indicate continuing small rises in numbers of new AIDS cases in the mid-1990s. But Chin's remarks on the epidemic in the developing world received gloomy assent from his audience. While there were some listeners who might have disputed his prediction that, ten years hence, 90 per cent of AIDS cases would be located in the developing world, their disagreements would have centred on his optimistic forecasts for the course of the epidemic in the developed world; his gloomy forecasts for the course of the developing world epidemic have met with little disagreement.

It has long been recognised that the epidemic in the developing world has a different character from that in the developed world. The World Health Organisation distinguishes between, on the one hand 'Pattern-I' countries where sufferers are largely male and either men who have sex with men or else injecting drug users, and on the other hand, 'Pattern II' countries with relatively more female sufferers and a distinctive pattern of largely heterosexual transmission. Initially, these Pattern II countries were located in Africa and the Caribbean, but this pattern is now also being found in certain Asian countries, notably India and Thailand. Even a low level of heterosexual transmission of HIV in the populous countries of Asia will greatly increase current global numbers of sufferers.

This chapter begins with a description of Pattern II transmission found in some African countries, with particular emphasis on the 'core groups' hypothesis as an explanation of rapid epidemic spread. The emphasis will be epidemiological and descriptive, with only incidental reference to continuing HIV-related risk behaviour and risk reduction (the sociological analysis of risk behaviour being the main focus of Chapter 4). It is suggested that the 'core groups' hypothesis is subject to local and regional modification due to local and regional differences in sexual behaviours and cultural meanings, and that these differences may themselves be important in understanding epidemiological variations in HIV spread. Following examination of the 'core groups' hypothesis, consideration is given to three factors whose roles in the Third World epidemic are currently uncertain but potentially important: sex tourism, drug trafficking and male prostitution. The chapter concludes with speculations on future trends: consideration of whether an African-style epidemic is on the cards in the very different developing world societies of South Asia and South America; and consideration of whether the African epidemic can still be halted by intervention campaigns targeted at 'core groups'.

The African epidemic

There is still no such thing as an African epidemic of HIV in the pan-continental sense. Some countries have reported very few AIDS cases to the World Health Organisation: Algeria – 138 cases; Eritrea – 372 cases (Table 2.1). WHO estimates of the spread of HIV in sub-Saharan Africa up to the end of 1988 showed that just nine countries, with only one-sixth of the local population in the region, accounted for two-thirds of the estimated numbers of HIV cases (Sato et al., 1989). Moreover, there are two distinct viral epidemics – an epidemic of HIV-1, concentrated in Central and East Africa but spilling out elsewhere, and an epidemic of HIV-2 in parts of West Africa. Of course, an absence of *reported* cases may reflect an absence of epidemiological investigation or ineffectual official reporting systems: in 1988 WHO estimated that some African nations were under-reporting by a factor of ten (Chin and Mann, 1988).

There remain some areas of the continent where the virus is currently completely absent or present only at very low levels of prevalence, for example among the pygmy peoples of Cameroon (Louis et al., 1993). But other areas which were until recently almost free of the epidemic are now reporting greatly increased prevalences: in Ethiopia the prevalence of HIV-1 among military recruits rose from 0.075 per cent in 1986 to 2.6 per cent in 1991 – a thirty-four-fold increase in five years (Kefenie et al., 1992).

The pan-African epidemic is a popular and media 'representation' of the epidemic, akin to earlier representations of 'The Gay Plague'. Kitzinger and Miller (1992) have combined content analyses of British TV and press reporting of the epidemic with 'focus group' techniques designed to elicit audience understandings of media reports from a range of British audience panels (pensioners, prison officers, male prostitutes, office cleaners, etc.). The researchers showed how audience images of a diseased population could be linked to media representations which conflated the particular and the pan-continental, for example studio backgrounds of the African continent in silhouette cut to shots of individual black sufferers. Even that notable social history of the epidemic, Randy Shilts's *And the Band Played On* (Shilts, 1987), which documented so carefully the various and changing responses to the epidemic of the American gay community, has portrayed the African experience of the disease in terms which are frankly phantasmagoric.

Taking first the HIV-2 epidemic, it has been suggested that this virus

Table 2.1   *Reported world AIDS cases to 30 June 1994*

World total: 985,119

Europe: 115,668	Africa: 331,376
Austria: 1,150	Botswana: 1,415
Belgium: 1,603	Burkina Faso: 4,193
Denmark: 1,411	Burundi: 7,225
France: 30,003	Cameroon: 3,072
Germany: 11,179	Central African Rep.: 3,730
Italy: 21,770	Chad: 1,523
Netherlands: 3,055	Congo: 6,393
Portugal: 18,011	Cote d'Ivoire: 18,670
Romania: 2,736	Ethiopia: 12,958
Spain: 24,202	Ghana: 11,629
Sweden: 1,001	Kenya: 30,126
Switzerland: 3,662	Malawi: 31,857
UK: 9,025	Mali: 1,874
(others >1,000)	Namibia: 5,101
	Nigeria: 1,148
Americas: 523,777	Rwanda: 10,706
Argentina: 3,904	South Africa: 3,210
Bahamas: 1,389	Tanzania: 38,719
Brazil: 49,312	Togo: 3,472
Canada: 9,511	Uganda: 43,875
Colombia: 4,583	Zaire: 22,747
Dominican Rep.: 2,353	Zambia: 29,734
Haiti: 4,967	Zimbabwe: 27,905
Honduras: 3,473	(others <1,000)
Mexico: 18,353	
Peru: 1,068	Asia: 8,968
Trinidad: 1,545	Thailand: 5,654
USA: 411,907	(others <1,000)
Venezuela: 3,511	
(others <1,000)	Oceania: 5,330
	Australia: 4,727
	(others <1,000)

Source: WHO cumulative case reports at 30.6.94

may be less infectious than HIV-1 (Pepin et al., 1991; Wilkins et al., 1993; Ricard et al., 1994). However, it has also been suggested that HIV-2 may have a longer latency period (the asymptomatic period prior to the development of full-blown AIDS), so that lesser infectiousness may be partly counter-balanced by a longer period during which infection may take place. Certainly, there is evidence that the virus is now widely distributed: although only identified in 1986 (Clavel et al., 1986), it appears to have been present in some localities in Africa since at least the late 1960s. Thus, Ancelle-Park et al. (1987) reported the development of AIDS in a Portuguese couple resident in France with no history of injecting drug use, or blood transfusions, or recent sexual intercourse outside marriage. However, the man had done his military service in Portuguese West Africa (now Guinea-Bissau) from 1966 to 1969, where he had been treated for an unidentified sexually transmitted disease. By 1990 HIV-2 was being identified in many locations remote from West Africa, for example among injecting drug users in the American Pacific Coast city of Seattle (Harris et al., 1990).

General population studies of the prevalence of HIV-2 are few in number. A 1988 population survey of the Gambia (host to a research unit of the British Medical Research Council) showed an overall prevalence of 1.6 per cent for HIV-2 and 0.1 per cent for HIV-1 (Wilkins et al., 1991). A team from the same research unit also undertook a survey of a rural area of Guinea-Bissau (population 7,000) where the numbers of persons with full-blown AIDS indicated that the virus had been present for some time; the prevalence of HIV-2 was in excess of 15 per cent in some age groups (Ricard et al., 1994). There is also some evidence that, at least among those segments of the population where HIV-2 is already established, it is the more recent import, HIV-1, which is spreading fastest. A repeat cross-sectional study of prostitutes in the Gambia in 1988 and 1989 showed the prevalence of HIV-2 to have remained unchanged at 25 per cent, while the prevalence of HIV-1 rose from 1 per cent to 7 per cent in the same year (Pepin et al., 1991). Similar results have been obtained from repeat cross-sectional studies of Senegalese prostitutes (M'Boup et al., 1990).

The epidemiology of HIV-1 is better documented. Indeed, a senior civil servant has disclosed that the trigger which led to the British government's AIDS information campaigns was the circulation within the higher echelons of the then Department of Health and Social Security in 1986 of an early paper indicating substantial levels of HIV infection in urban areas of Zambia: it was the spectre of a heterosexual epidemic in Britain on a similar scale to that apparently occurrent in parts of Africa which jolted the Conservative government into uncharacteristic state intervention.

In the event, some (but not all) of the apocalyptic predictions of the mid-1980s have remained unjustified. As Jonathan Mann, former head of WHO's Global Programme on AIDS, has pointed out (Mann, 1991) the current situation is quite a complex one with some urban areas having apparently achieved near-stable HIV prevalences (for example, Kinshasa in Zaire – Quinn et al., 1986) while others show continuing rapid increases (for example, Abidjan on the Ivory Coast – Soro et al., 1990). Nevertheless, even if HIV prevalence were to stabilise at current levels, the scale of the epidemic would still be literally decimating: among women attending antenatal clinics at Lilongwe and Blantyre in

Malawi HIV prevalence was 10 per cent in 1989 (Guertler et al., 1989); unlinked anonymous testing of women attending a range of Kenyan antenatal clinics in 1991 produced an overall 10.1 per cent HIV prevalence (Mboya, 1993).

Uncertainty remains over the future spread of the disease in rural areas and some commentators have hoped that supposed urban/rural differences in sexual behaviour might keep rural prevalence rates comparatively low. However, a prevalence rate of 8.5 per cent among adults in a rural region of Uganda (Mulder et al., 1991) suggests that this may be a pious hope. Certainly, many rural communities that abut important highways or navigable rivers are already areas of high prevalence. HIV prevalences in the Mwanza Project in north-western Tanzania varied between those of the town at 11.8 per cent and a rural area at 2.8 per cent. However a rural area beside an important highway had a prevalence of 7.3 per cent in 1990 (Hayes, 1991).

Differences in the social patterning of infection are particularly important in relation to the transmission dynamics of the epidemic. Mathematical models of epidemic spread lay stress on the pivotal importance of that small minority of persons who are very sexually active (Anderson and May, 1988). Sexually transmitted disease epidemics are driven, not by the sexual behaviour (safe or unsafe) of the majority, but by that of a very active minority: a case of the tail wagging the dog.

Parallels have been drawn between the HIV/AIDS epidemic and epidemics of gonorrhoea in Western societies, where the role of 'core groups' (Yorke et al., 1978) is thought to be of crucial importance in sustaining the epidemic. Plummer and his associates (Plummer et al., 1991) have pointed out that HIV is not very readily transmitted. The *average* transmission frequency of HIV-1 during one episode of sexual intercourse is, according to WHO estimates, somewhere between one in a thousand and one in a hundred. A multi-centre European Community study, following up transmission between couples with discordant HIV statuses, has suggested similarly low transmission probabilities: an average transmission rate of one per thousand exposures (95 per cent confidence interval – 0.5 to 1.7) – de Vincenzi (1994). Since we must assume that, in the absence of new therapeutic advances, the great majority of those infected with HIV-1 will eventually die, then for the virus to remain in circulation an infected person must have sex with one person between a hundred and a thousand times, or else have sex with between a hundred and a thousand new partners. As we shall see, very little is known about the sociology of sexual behaviour but it seems highly unlikely that many persons will report hundreds (or thousands!) of different sexual partners. And yet the speed of epidemic spread in Africa suggests that this kind of rapid partner change must have occurred. The answer to this conundrum, according to Plummer and his colleagues, lies partly in the role of 'core groups' – small numbers of highly sexually active individuals with large numbers of partners who mix with individuals who might otherwise be deemed at low risk of infection.

This heterogeneous mixing of 'core groups' with less sexually active partners explains another potentially puzzling feature of the epidemic, that of why 'saturation' (as it is somewhat chillingly termed) has not occurred: if the highly sexually active mix very largely with partners who are also highly sexually active, then most of those partners will also eventually be infected and new cases of infection will be few – 'saturation' will have occurred. As we have already seen, although prevalence has apparently stabilized in a few local African populations, there is no evidence of such saturation having occurred in many others. Continuing rapid epidemic spread depends not just on rapid partner change, but also on the heterogenous mixing of infected individuals with partners from different social backgrounds and different geographical areas.

Readers will already have surmised that female prostitutes would constitute one such 'core group', a dismaying identification for those who deplore the vilification of women who are frequently already the victims of exploitation and discrimination and who are frequently driven by want and destitution to that behaviour known euphemistically as 'rapid partner change'. However, it should be stressed here that there is no necessity for epidemiology to collude with punitive responses to prostitution. Rather, the recognition of the pivotal role of prostitution in HIV spread in many African countries may be the precursor of intervention programmes of great benefit to the prostitute population (Plummer and his colleagues have demonstrated the benefits of such programmes even in narrow economic terms – Moses et al., 1991).

It is certain that HIV prevalences are high in many African prostitute populations. Repeated studies of over a thousand prostitutes living in a low income area of Nairobi (Kenya) have shown HIV prevalences of 80 per cent and over since 1988 (Moses et al., 1991). And other African studies have found a strong association between AIDS in heterosexual males and a history of sex with prostitutes (Clumeck et al., 1985). A prostitute, once infected by a client, may transmit that infection to other clients who, in turn, may infect their wives and girlfriends: in a pre-AIDS survey of female attenders at a Nairobi venereal disease clinic 56 per cent of the women were reported to have been infected by their husbands (cited in Day, 1988).

Colonialism and neo-colonialism have substituted cash crops for much subsistence agriculture while providing labouring jobs in the towns and the mines, creating a large, male, migrant labour force. This massive social dislocation seems to have produced somewhat various consequences in respect of sexual behaviour. Among the Luo people it is commonplace for men to have two wives – one to run the home farm in the husband's native village and one to run the house in the town where the husband labours (Parkin, 1978).

In some African cities, migration patterns have created substantial sexual imbalances in the population; these imbalances create opportunities for substantial prostitute populations while alternative economic earning possibilities for urban women may be very limited. Day (1988) distinguishes between two types of Nairobi prostitution – 'wazi wazi' and 'malaya'. While 'wazi wazi' prostitution is the sale of sex alone, 'malaya' prostitution (often practised by Kikuyu women) involves the sale of sex, food and lodging and is not readily distinguishable from formal marriage, frequently involving associations with clients lasting several years. In the Gambia, in contrast, Western-style prostitution, based on bars, is practised by women who are themselves largely migrants from neighbouring Senegal and (less commonly) Guinea-Bissau (Pickering et al., 1992).

Plummer and his colleagues have suggested that a second 'core group' is formed by long-distance lorry drivers; they may inter-link with the prostitute 'core group' by acting as highly geographically mobile clients spreading HIV along the highways among each of the local prostitute populations, as well as casual girlfriends (see Carswell, 1987). However, some studies have shown that some prostitute populations are themselves highly geographically mobile. An anthropological study of the isolated camps for the commercial fishermen of Lake Kariba (in Zimbabwe) showed prostitutes making frequent visits to the camps when their business in the cities was slack, often paying for their lorry or boat transport with sexual services; 82 per cent of the fishermen interviewed had been clients of prostitutes, 60 per cent in the previous month (Wilson et al., 1991). Many of those Gambian prostitutes studied by Pickering and her colleagues travelled not just between towns and back to their home villages but also moved around Sene-Gambian rural areas prostituting at the weekly village markets (Pickering et al., 1992).

Unless safer sex is practised, these highly sexually active 'core groups' of women and men (and there may be other 'core groups' besides the lorry drivers) are likely to be comparatively 'efficient' transmitters of HIV. This is because 'core group' members are more likely than the general population to be infected with other sexually transmitted diseases: these diseases, such as chancroid with its characteristic genital ulceration, are thought to increase substantially the likelihood of HIV transmission. Genital ulceration increases the likelihood of both male-to-female and female-to-male transmission; non-ulcerative STDs (chlamydial infection, gonorrhoea, and trichomoniasis) increase transmission from male to female. The strengths of these co-factor effects are not known accurately, but for genital ulceration the potential for the enhancement of transmission appears to be substantial, particularly for female-to-male transmission (Hayes, 1993; Laga et al., 1991). Nevertheless, as will be seen in Chapter 4, the importance of 'core group' HIV transmission is likely to vary between different African cultures. Some African societies which offer more economic opportunities to women (for example, access to land) may thus allow women the freedom to take more sexual partners; the consequent greater equality in sexual mixing patterns between men and women reduces the relative importance of prostitute–client contacts and allows a limited role for 'core groups' in epidemic spread.

Outside of the 'core groups', information on the social patterning of the epidemic is fragmentary for most African countries. Media coverage of the deaths of the socially prominent, such as the son of Kenneth Kaunda, the former Zambian president, have fostered the impression that prevalence is greatest among the urban elite, but this may be misleading. Certainly, research in rural Uganda shows the comparatively well-off (as measured by house construction, land tenure, cattle ownership and household possessions) have only half the prevalence rate of the rural poor (Mulder et al., 1991). Elsewhere, in Tanzania, associations have been found between positive HIV status and travel and marital status, with higher rates among the widowed, separated and divorced (Hayes, 1991). Particular occupations, notably soldiering (as in Rwanda), have also been associated with HIV positivity.

The speed by which epidemics spread is measured epidemiologically by the 'doubling time', the period of time in which the numbers of infected persons double. In the earliest stages of an epidemic the doubling time is shortest; later on the doubling time gradually lengthens, due to factors such as 'saturation' and differential susceptibility to infection. In areas of Africa where HIV-1 has only recently become established, such as West Africa, the doubling time is relatively short (fourteen months in the Gambia – Wilkins et al., 1991), supporting WHO calculations of further large increases in African AIDS cases in the 1990s. But James Chin's estimation, at the Florence conference, that only 10 per cent of AIDS cases by the year 2000 would be in the developed world, depends not just on the continuing African epidemic but also on rapid epidemic spread in other areas of the developing world, especially in Latin America and Asia. It is to these areas that we now turn.

Latin America and Asia

South America has some claim to be the forgotten continent of the AIDS epidemic. After the USA, the country with the greatest number of *reported* AIDS cases is not an African country: it is Brazil, with 49,312 reported cases as at 30 June 1994, compared to 43,875 in Uganda (WHO Weekly Epidemiological Record, 1 July 1994). This has occurred despite a probable considerable degree of under-reporting of cases as sufferers go undiagnosed, either because their poverty excludes them from medical care, or because their symptoms are confused with those of tropical diseases long endemic in Brazil. WHO estimated the total numbers of HIV-positive persons in South and Central America in 1993 at between one and one and a half million.

The social patterning of the Latin American epidemic fits neither that of the developed world, nor that of Africa, a fact recognised by its designation by WHO as a 'Pattern I/II' epidemic. The earliest reported cases were among homosexual men: in Brazil, the first AIDS deaths, occurring in 1983, were all among homosexual men who had previously spent some time in New York (Trevisan, cited in Parker, 1987). However, heterosexual transmission rapidly assumed greater numerical importance.

Although the first Brazilian cases were found among the affluent middle classes, the virus is now found primarily among the poor. It has been detected, for example, among the 'street children', the tatterdemalion juveniles mainly known outside Latin America as the targets of vigilante death squads. It is unclear when HIV was first established among the continent's injecting drug users, but it seems likely that it was later than in the USA and Europe. However, in the WHO cross-national study of HIV infection among injecting drug users involving eleven different participating international centres (WHO Collaborative Study Group, 1993), HIV prevalence among injectors in São Paulo State (59 per cent) was higher than prevalence among injectors in centres such as London (12 per cent) and even New York (46 per cent) and Bangkok (34 per cent). Whether or not HIV has flowed backwards along the drug trafficking routes to the cocaine sources in Colombia, Peru and Bolivia remains largely uninvestigated, although local consumption of cocaine has traditionally been by chewing and smoking, rather than injection.

The different pattern of epidemic spread in Latin American countries may be attributed to distinctive sexual practices. The ethnographers, Parker (1987) and Perlongher (1987), have pointed out that the homosexual/heterosexual dichotomy used in epidemiological analyses is culturally alien to Brazil, where the central distinction is between masculine 'atividade' (activity) and feminine 'passividade' (passivity), between those who 'comem', who symbolically consume their male or female partners by taking the active penetrative role during intercourse, and those (male or female) who 'dao', who are passively penetrated by their active partners (Parker, 1987: 160–161). This suggests – in First World terms – a relatively greater prevalence of bisexuality. Indeed, more than 20 per cent of AIDS patients being treated in Rio de Janeiro in 1986 were classed as bisexuals, a much greater proportion than in the USA (Costa, cited by Parker, 1987). Moreover, this Brazilian active/passive dichotomony is itself overlain and blurred by an erotic playfulness in which public norms of sexual conduct are zestfully transgressed in private. This is the erotic ideal of 'sacanagem' (Parker, 1987) with its piquant role reversals and its code of 'fazendo tudo' (i.e. doing everything), its broad repertoire of sexual practices and relative emphasis on both oral sex and anal intercourse. This is an erotic culture of great richness: Perlongher, for example, recorded fifty-six different names for the 'miche', the male prostitute hustlers of São Paulo (Perlongher, 1987). It is a culture only dimly and inadequately perceived by European and American eyes via sanitised Hollywood images of 'carnival'. Small wonder that Parker complains that Euro-American epidemiology has inadequately conceptualised the transmission dynamics of HIV infection in Brazil.

The complex patterning of sexual behaviour in Brazil is reflected to some degree in Mexico, where same-sex encounters may occur extensively (particularly prior to marriage) without compromising the heterosexual identity of the active (penetrative) partner, and where anal intercourse is sometimes reported among engaged couples to preserve vaginal virginity (Carrier, 1989). Similarly detailed reports are unavailable from other Latin American countries but Boulton and Weatherburn (1990) surmise that bisexual behaviour (without bisexual *identification*) may be widespread in these countries, with anal intercourse commonly practised with both male and female passive partners.

Sex tourism may also be playing a part in Latin American HIV transmission: it is thought that a substantial proportion of the massive numbers of foreign visitors to the Brazilian Carnival may have sex during their visit, but hard data are lacking. The Dominican Republic and Mexico are sex tourism destinations for North Americans.

Sex tourism is also a probable feature of HIV transmission in Southern Asia. If South America is characterisable as the forgotten continent of the HIV/AIDS epidemic, then Asia is the continent waiting for the epidemic to happen. Recent reports of epidemic spread in India, Indonesia, Thailand and elsewhere have led to speculations among epidemiologists that Asia may overtake Africa by the end of the 1990s as the continent with largest numbers of HIV cases, although even as late as mid-1988 the total number of Asian cases was estimated at well under 100,000 compared to Africa's 2.5 million (Sato et al., 1989). In 1993, in contrast, WHO estimated more than 2 million HIV cases in South and South East Asia.

At each of the great annual AIDS conferences, among all the many hundreds of papers and poster presentations, there seems always to be one paper which stands out from the others, galvanising the delegates and exciting the attendant newspaper reporters. At the Washington conference in 1987 it was the report of a wholly unexpected epidemic of HIV among Edinburgh drug injectors. At the fifth conference in Montreal in 1989 it was the report that the prevalence of HIV infection among Bangkok drug injectors had risen from 1 per cent in late 1987 to over 40 per cent in early 1989 (Vanichseni et al., 1989). This staggering increase indicated a doubling time for the epidemic of only around three months. Further investigation suggests the rapidity of spread may have been due to particular local injecting equipment sharing practices: it was commonplace for the dealer to supply the injector with the 'works' and the 'hit', ready-prepared. The uncleaned 'works' would then be recovered and re-filled for the dealer's next customer – a form of serial anonymous sharing. Drug injecting in prison with shared works was also thought to be common.

The prevalence of HIV among Bangkok injectors now appears to have stabilised (Des Jarlais et al., 1991). However, at the 1990 AIDS conference in San Francisco further results were available, this time of attempts to establish HIV prevalence, not just among injecting drug users, but also among prisoners, male and female prostitutes, GUM (genito-urinary medicine) clinic attenders, antenatal clinic attenders and blood donors in fourteen different Thai provinces (Ungchusak et al., 1990). The results seemed to confirm the important role of equip-ment-sharing in prisons in that pre-release male prisoners had notably higher rates of HIV than newly admitted prisoners. But more impor-tantly the results showed that HIV was established much more widely than just among the drug-injecting population. Prevalence was very uneven between the different Thai provinces; however, rates among female prostitutes in brothels were as high as 44 per cent in one province (rates were lower among prostitutes who did not work in brothels). Rates among male GUM clinic attenders were as high as 10 per cent in one province. The rates among blood donors and antenatal clinic attenders might be thought to be those most representative of the general Thai population. Here too the data were alarming: as many as one in a hundred women attending clinics in one province were infected and the top provincial prevalence rate for blood donors was 3.7 per cent.

A full-scale epidemic of heterosexually transmitted HIV is now occurring in Thailand. Studies of HIV-positive male blood donors and male GUM clinic attenders found that 92 per cent of the infected blood donors and 80 per cent of the infected clinic attenders had engaged in no risk practices other than heterosexual contact (Kunanusont et al., 1991). It is unclear whether HIV infection spread from the drug-injecting population to the prostitute population: very few Thai drug injectors are women, and molecular epidemiologists have noted clear differences between genotypes drawn from virus isolates in the drug-injecting and prostitute populations, evidence suggestive of distinct but parallel epidemics. But once HIV was established in the prostitute population, heterosexual transmission was widespread, facilitated by a high prevalence of genital ulceration.

The Thai experience must be a matter of grave concern to those who fear an explosion of HIV infection among the multitudes of the Indian sub-continent. As in Africa, male Indian peasants have migrated to the cities in their search for employment. As in Africa, large numbers of female prostitutes (an estimated 10,000 in Madras alone) cater for this migrant population. HIV is already present both in Indian prostitute and in drug injector populations.

Up to March 1990 there were only 2,167 reports of HIV positivity in India and only 5 of these were of injecting drug users. However, in January 1991 there was a startling report in a professional journal of an HIV epidemic among drug injectors in Manipur in north-east India (Naik et al., 1991). Manipur borders the Golden Triangle of opium production and local heroin smugglers are known to journey frequently into Thailand. Because drug-injecting is widespread in Manipur (with an estimated 15,000 injectors), monitoring of possible HIV infection has been taking place since 1986. However, no cases of infection were found until late 1989. Subsequent spread has been rapid: prevalence among drug injectors was estimated in 1991 at 54 per cent. It has been suggested that there is a drug trafficking link between the Indian epidemic and the recent Nigerian epidemic, with a 9 per cent prevalence of HIV-1 among the high-class Nigerian prostitutes who consort with those Indian businessmen and drugs traffickers who are part of the Nigeria–India international trafficking link (Dada et al., 1993).

High levels of HIV infection have now been reported among drug injectors in the world's most populous country, China. In three rural counties in Yunnan Province, alongside the Burmese border, the prevalence of HIV among drug injectors is 49 per cent; among the wives of male drug injectors HIV prevalence is 10 per cent (Zheng et al., 1994).

There is no claimed link between the Indian drug injector and prostitute epidemic. The latter has shown rapid increases among some, but not all, Indian female prostitute populations. The prevalence of HIV among Bombay prostitutes increased from just 1 per cent in 1986 to 38 per cent in 1994; the Indian government's National AIDS Control Organisation estimates that the overall level of HIV infection among Indian prostitute women in 1994 was 7.5 per cent (cited in Shannuganaudan et al., 1994).

The possible role of sex tourism in epidemic spread is little researched and understood. If Thai police estimates are correct, that 60 per cent of foreign visitors are sex tourists, then Thailand has more than 2 million sex tourists a year, 100,000 of them from Britain. Interviews with German sex tourists in Thailand indicated that nearly half of the men (46 per cent) never wore condoms in their contacts with Thai women (Kleiber et al., 1991). In contrast, among those who reported contacts with prostitutes in Germany, the proportion who claimed never to wear condoms was only 12.5 per cent. These international differences in condom use are only partially attributable to the more limited bargaining power of Thai prostitutes. The men themselves did not, for the most part, see themselves as consorting with prostitutes, preferring to see their holiday sex as a romantic interlude: more than 40 per cent of the men claimed to have fallen in love with a Thai woman and 63 per cent had spent several days with their last Thai 'date'. The absence of a condom is seen as emblematic of intimacy and romance. Their Thai prostitutes collude in this romantic interpretation of their relationships, since the women consider it shameful not to show affection to their consorts.

Like Thailand, the Philippines developed a sex tourism industry in the Vietnam war, although the largest number of visitors now come from Japan. There were 76,000 British visitors in 1987, some of them seekers after 'catalogue' Filipino brides (500 of whom entered Britain in 1990 – *Independent*, 28 November 1991). HIV prevalence is currently low, but other sexually transmitted diseases are common and condom use is also low (Monzon et al., 1990; Bagasao et al., 1990a).

The Philippines is of course a Pacific rather than an Asian nation. Other Asian countries with a sex tourism industry are South Korea (mainly catering for Japanese visitors), Hong Kong, India (Goa) and Sri Lanka – Sri Lankan officials estimate that 10 per cent of foreign visitors have sex with Sri Lankan nationals during their stay (Panos Institute, 1989).

The degree to which sex tourism results in Third World epidemic spread will depend on the degree of local segregation of the sex industry: where prostitutes have both tourist and local clients, then epidemic spread is likely to be rapid. Detailed information is lacking but it seems that client overlap among Thai female prostitutes is quite limited, with women either working in bars and massage parlours patronised very largely by tourists, or else working mainly in establishments visited by their fellow nationals. Pickering and her colleagues (1992) report a similar segregation in the Gambia.

Patterns of sexual mixing may be different in respect of male prostitution. The practice of male prostitution varies enormously between and within different Third World countries (see Boulton and Weatherburn, 1990, for a brief overview). In some countries, however, there are substantial male prostitute populations who self-identify as heterosexual or bisexual, having commercial sexual relationships with men and private sexual relationships with women. Indeed, among the Brazilian 'miche' it is their macho self-image which constitutes their piquant attraction to their male clients: 'Normalement, les garçons de la nuit ne sont pas ou ne se considèrent pas des homosexuals et c'est dans ce refus, demandé par les clients eux-mêmes (qui cherchent des mecs qui ne soient pas homosexuels), qui se trouve une bonne partie de leur charme' (Perlongher, 1987: 8). In a study of 250 male prostitutes in the Philippines, 63 per cent were described by the authors as 'bisexual' (Bagasao et al., 1990). Among male street prostitutes in Rio de Janeiro HIV prevalence was 61 per cent; only 31 per cent of the HIV-positive respondents reported always using condoms with their private partners (Van Buuren and Longo, 1991).

The possible role of male prostitution in HIV transmission remains largely unresearched in both the developed world and the developing world, but what little that is known suggests that parallels between male and female prostitution may be misleading. Indeed, it may be misleading to treat male prostitution as a unitary phenomenon at all, since it has so many diverse manifestations: the role in epidemic transmission of the masculine Brazilian 'miche' may be quite different from that of his male prostitute colleague, the 'travesti' (transvestite). However, Cespedes and his colleagues (1992) have suggested that male prostitutes may be playing an unwitting 'core group' epidemiological role in the South American epidemic. This is a topic to which we shall return in later chapters.

Conclusion

It is clear that broad epidemiological patterns of HIV incidence and prevalence conceal considerable local and regional differences in sexual behaviours and cultural meanings – differences in the extent and nature of female prostitution, differences in the economic position of women, differences in the construction of masculine identities, differences in the nature and extent of male prostitution, drug-injecting and sex tourism. These various local differences in culture and practice appear to modify, rather than demolish, the 'core groups' hypothesis. It seems that 'core groups' have indeed played a part in HIV spread, but this part has been subject to considerable local and regional variation in both nature and importance. It is even possible that phenomena such as variations in the speed of epidemic spread may be explicable by reference to how far local cultural practices may be locally modifying 'core group' influences.

It is worthwhile reiterating earlier cautionary comments on statistical representations of the epidemic. Statistics are not value-free: the ways in which statistical data are collected, aggregated and presented embody various latent assumptions of the statistician and invoke certain assumptions in the reader. Consider the collection and presentation of HIV prevalence data from female prostitutes: it may be an assumption of the reader that high HIV prevalence rates among women prostitutes are indicative of the women's role in epidemic spread. This can be seen in the sensationalist media reporting of research findings on prostitution in the developed world, where findings of HIV infection among women prostitutes have produced lurid tabloid headlines. Of course, high prevalences of HIV are perfectly consistent with low rates of disease transmission, provided the infected persons are practising safer sex. Something like this has in fact occurred in parts of the developed world, where enhanced rates of HIV among women prostitutes as a consequence of injecting drug use do not appear to have produced a client epidemic, because of widespread condom use by prostitutes (see Chapters 3 and 4).

Consideration of Third World HIV/AIDS prevalence data alone may lead to over-pessimistic assumptions about the course of the Third World epidemic, since even where existing levels of infection are high, future infections may be low: much depends on the behaviour of the infected and their partners. Since the epidemiological 'core groups' have been pivotal in epidemic spread, they may equally be pivotal in epidemic prevention. If 'core group' members (whether infected or uninfected) can be assisted and induced to practise safer sex, then overall new cases of infection will be progressively reduced, because infected persons outside the 'core groups' will experience limited partner change and because the chances of transmitting HIV to one of these partners may be only one or two in a thousand sexual acts. Although there may continue to be further infections in the short term, as those previous casual partners of 'core group' members transmit the infection to their regular partners, a successful intervention campaign targeted at 'core group' members is likely to reduce dramatically new infections in the medium term, even in areas of East and Central Africa where the disease is now widespread. Deprived of a continuing input of new infections among the casual partners of 'core group' members, the argument runs, the natural transmission dynamics of the epidemic will ensure an eventual dwindling of new cases. A similar argument applies to the treatment of other sexually transmitted diseases among 'core group' members: successful treatment of other STDs which amplify the transmissibility of HIV will itself serve to reduce rates of HIV transmission, in addition to the impact of moves towards safer commercial sex.

It may be objected that this strategy of prevention campaigns targeted closely at 'core groups' is too dependent on fragile assumptions about the limited transmissibility of the virus. Caution counsels that we know too little of the behaviour of the virus, too little of the biological determinants of differential infectiousness and differential susceptibility to infection, too little of the role of genetics and of possible co-factors such as other sexually transmitted diseases. If HIV should prove more readily transmissible than we suspect, at least among certain more infectious and/or more susceptible sub-sections of the population, then an intervention strategy targeted at 'core groups' could be a flop.

Nevertheless, a 'core groups' intervention strategy may represent the best hope for public health in many African countries. Vaccines, 'therapeutic' vaccines and pharmacological treatments, once developed and available, would be well beyond the purchasing power of Third World countries whose total per capita health care budgets would not cover even the issue of free condoms. Numerous commentators have questioned whether there will be sufficient political will in the developed world to provide the massive aid necessary to make expensive new vaccines and treatments available to developing world populations. Under these circumstances, the low cost of the 'core groups' intervention strategy may be a decisive advantage.

The various components of such an intervention strategy will be considered in more detail in the final chapter. It needs to be pointed out, however, that some aspects of the strategy are more readily accomplished than others. It may be a relatively straightforward matter, for example, to provide effective treatment to prostitutes for other sexually transmitted diseases (such as chancroid) which may facilitate HIV spread. It may be a straightforward matter to provide the same women with free condoms. But it may be much more difficult to ensure that the condoms are widely used, where clients are disinclined. The effectiveness of the 'core groups' intervention strategy depends, not just on the transmissibility of the virus, but also on the health education approach used to promote behaviour change. It depends, in other words, on an understanding of the sociology (or the anthropology) of HIV transmission as well as on the epidemiology of HIV transmission. This is a topic to which we shall return.

If a 'core groups' intervention strategy seems the best hope for those countries where prevalence is already high, then it is still more surely the best hope for prevention in those Third World countries where the epidemic is not already entrenched. The evidence reviewed here suggests that the range of potential 'core groups' may be wider than those identified in Africa. Drug injectors and male prostitutes may possibly both act as epidemiological 'core groups' – the evidence is unclear and their influence will be locally variable. Drug trafficking is not the only possible route for the introduction of HIV into Third World countries, sex tourism being another alternative. Male prostitution may be of more importance locally than female prostitution, since male prostitutes may have male, tourist, commercial, sexual partners and local, female, private, sexual partners. Among Third World female prostitutes, in contrast, those catering for sex tourists may not normally cater for local casual partners as well.

These issues – drug trafficking, sex tourism, Third World male prostitution – have been little researched and are poorly understood. There is a danger that distinctive local cultural practices may be misinterpreted by developed world observers, as Parker has argued that Brazilian sexual practices have been misunderstood by observers used to a clear-cut homosexual/heterosexual division in sexual identification and practice. Local programmes of intervention and prevention will require local cultural knowledge if they are to be effective. To echo an earlier point, the sociology and anthropology of HIV transmission may be the crucial tools of epidemiology and public health.

3

The Epidemic of HIV Infection
in the Developed World

The government information campaigns on HIV/AIDS that were launched in 1986 in developed countries such as Britain and Australia were essentially a response to the African epidemic rather than to the epidemics already occurring within their own borders. At that time reliable commercial blood tests for the virus had just been developed and the results of the first tests from population samples were becoming available. As discussed in the last chapter, some of the early African studies indicated the literal decimation of local populations, with one in ten of some urban populations already infected with the virus. It was the attempt to forestall a widespread, African-style, heterosexual epidemic in the West that led the British government to adopt unprecedented health education measures, such as mailshots to every household in the land. As Shilts (1987) has pointed out in his social history of the American epidemic, it took the threat of a heterosexual epidemic to galvanise governments to intervene in respect of a public health threat that was already decimating gay men, injecting drug users and haemophiliacs. This has led to some sardonic commentaries from the gay community.

The feared, decimating heterosexual epidemic has not, to date, materialised in the developed world. As we shall see, this probably has to do with the more limited importance in developed countries of African-style 'core groups' and the absence of co-factors facilitating transmission, particularly the comparative rarity of untreated sexually transmitted diseases causing genital ulceration. It probably has little to do with government information campaigns.

The heterosexual epidemic that has occurred thus far is not in the African pattern; it is an epidemic of so-called 'secondary transmission' – transmission to the heterosexual partners of infected bisexuals, haemophiliacs and (most importantly) injecting drug users. Primary transmission, if one may so term infection from a person him/herself infected from heterosexual intercourse, has been recorded among British nationals comparatively infrequently. Of course, further cases of primary transmission can be expected as secondary transmission becomes more common, as the infectiousness of HIV-positive individuals increases following their progression to ARC (AIDS-related complex) and AIDS, and as heterosexual mixing occurs with sexual partners from those parts of the developing world where rapid HIV transmission is occurring. Nevertheless, reportage of Western heterosexual transmission here and in subsequent chapters will primarily be concerned with secondary transmission. However, I will address first of all epidemic spread in those two transmission categories that account for the great majority of HIV cases in the developed world – men who have sex with men, and injecting drug users (Table 3.1).

The epidemiological term 'transmission category' should not be confused with the discredited and stigmatising term 'risk group'. No one is at risk of infection because of their membership of a group, only because they engage in certain risk practices. Injecting drug users are not at risk because they inject drugs: they are only at risk if they share their injecting equipment. The American government agency, the Centers for Disease Control, which first developed the internationally used HIV transmission categories for the epidemiological differentiation of infection routes, employed the term 'homosexual and bisexual'; 'men who have sex with men' is the term preferred here, since not all these individuals will self-identify as 'gay' or 'bisexual'. We have already noted the cultural estrangement of Brazilian and Mexican men from labels such as 'gay' or 'bisexual', for example, while being ready to act as insertor partners in same-sex relations. Most Glasgow male prostitutes reported that the majority of their clients were married men (Bloor et al., 1991a), many of whom would deny or conceal a gay or bisexual identification.

References to HIV infection in this chapter will refer exclusively to HIV-1, since HIV-2, although now identified as present in many parts of the developed world, is still very uncommon. In the UK, for example, only 34 cases had been identified up to 1993; many of these cases had African connections and are likely to have contracted their infections when abroad.

Table 3.1 *Reported UK HIV-1 cases by transmission category, to 30 June 1994 (22,101 cases)*

Transmission category	Male	Female	Unknown	Total
Men who have sex with men (MWHSWM)	13,381	–	–	13,381
Injecting drug use	1,775	809	4	2,588
MWHSWM and injecting drug use	298	–	–	298
Sexual intercourse between men and women	1,642	1,877	5	3,524
Blood and blood products [gender not stated]				1,383
Other/undetermined	674	221	32	927

Source: Public Health Laboratory Service, 1994

Men who have sex with men

This is the transmission category with the largest number of reported HIV cases in England and Wales, in most Northern European countries (*not* Scotland, or Ireland, or Southern Europe, where injecting drug users are the most numerous category), in Australasia and, of course, in North America. Similar preponderances occur in respect of reported AIDS cases. In the USA alone, up to June 1993, there were 172,085 reported AIDS cases among men who had sex with men (55 per cent of all adult US AIDS cases), with an additional 19,557 AIDS cases among men who both had sex with men and were injecting drug users (reported by US Centers for Disease Control and Prevention). In the UK, up to 31 December 1993, 6,318 of the total of 7,850 reported AIDS cases were among men who had sex with men, with an additional 134 cases among men who both had sex with men and were injecting drug users (Public Health Laboratory Service, 1994).

The first clinical report of pneumocystis pneumonia deaths among gay men in Los Angeles appeared in 1981 (Gottlieb et al., 1981) and the earliest epidemiological investigators were concerned, of course, with establishing modes of disease transmission. However, once the responsible viral agent had been isolated and once tests for antibodies to the virus were available, it was possible to test retrospectively blood samples from studies of gay men conducted in the 1970s and early 1980s, notably those of trials of hepatitis B vaccines (for example Van Griensven et al., 1989). It became clear that rates of new HIV infections had already been high among some local populations of American gay men in the late 1970s: Stevens et al. (1986) retrospectively recorded an annual seroconversion rate in New York in 1979 of 5.5 per cent. These incidence rates continued to climb in the early 1980s but then peaked and began to fall in the United States in 1984 (Centers for Disease Control, 1987). By 1986 and 1987 evidence of very low rates of new infections was being supplied by studies of gay men on three different continents.

Some caution is advised here. Many of these studies were of clinic samples, usually samples of gay men attending genito-urinary medicine clinics. Falls in HIV incidence were inferred from near stability (or even a fall) in annual prevalence rates among clinic attenders. There are two related methodological problems with such studies. Firstly, clinic samples are not representative of all men who have sex with men and are likely to over-represent 'fast-lane' gay men with previous histories of sexually transmitted diseases. And secondly, these 'fast-lane' gay men may be most strongly represented in the earliest years of such clinic studies, with a consequential inflation of early annual prevalence rates. Thus, Johnson and Gill comment of a reported *fall* in annual

HIV prevalence rates at a west London clinic (from 32 per cent in 1984 to 21 per cent in 1987 – Evans et al., 1989) that one explanation for such figures is that 'as time moves on, clinics are simply testing a lower risk population. Those at highest risk have already tested positive and therefore been removed from subsequent estimates of prevalence' (Johnson and Gill, 1989: 158).

Those studies that have attempted to recruit representative samples of men who have sex with men are thus worthy of particular attention. One such is that of a cohort of over a thousand single men aged 25 to 54 years living in a known gay area of San Francisco (Winkelstein et al., 1988). In this study annual HIV seroconversion rates dropped considerably from 18 per cent per annum in the early 1980s. Although the annual rate was still rather high at 4 per cent in 1986, seroconversions continued to fall and by the last six months of 1987 they were down to an 'annualized' rate of 0.7 per cent. The authors believe that this low rate of infection is 'unlikely to be attributable to selection bias of study participants. A more likely explanation is the decline in the prevalence of . . . anal intercourse' (Winkelstein et al., 1988: 1474).

The topic of changes in the risk practices of men who have sex with men is one that will be returned to in Chapter 4. Nevertheless, it is clear from the above San Francisco study and from other studies that have attempted to recruit non-clinic samples of gay men (for example, Project Sigma in England and Wales [Davies et al., 1993a] and the Macquarrie University study in Australia [Kippax et al., 1993]), that there have been very substantial falls in reports of unsafe sex in the 1980s. For example, in the San Francisco study reports of receptive anal intercourse with two or more partners in the previous six months had fallen by 80 per cent between 1984 and 1987. Further confirmation of this behaviour change comes from falls in rates of rectal gonorrhoea. Although rectal gonorrhoea can be transmitted in various ways (see Tomlinson et al., 1991a) it is undoubtedly strongly associated with receptive anal intercourse. At one London hospital rates of male rectal gonorrhoea fell 53 per cent between 1983/84 and 1986 (Gellan and Ison, 1986). Johnson and Gill (1989) have also suggested that falls in England and Wales in new cases among males of syphilis and hepatitis B may also be linked with changes in gay men's sexual behaviour.

There comes a point in every epidemic of sexually transmitted disease when the transmission dynamics of the epidemic will themselves produce a fall in the number of new cases, and near-stability in prevalence will be achieved. This may occur because of 'saturation', because the epidemic is so far advanced that most of the partners of the infected are themselves already infected. It may occur because of differential mixing, because those first infected choose their partners from a limited social group and have little contact with the uninfected. It may occur because infection is transmitted first among the most sexually active; their subsequent mortality means that the epidemic will continue to spread at a lower rate since it is now concentrated among the less sexually active. Or, a more likely scenario, a fall in disease incidence may occur because of some combination of two or three of these factors.

This is not to belittle the importance of sexual behaviour change within the gay community in arresting epidemic spread, a change in behaviour of arresting speed and magnitude, and a change which was achieved by local gay communities prior to belated government information campaigns. However, the precise role of these behaviour changes in epidemic transmission remains unclear. Certainly the mathematical modelling that has been conducted to date indicates that the impact on the magnitude of the epidemic is greatest when it occurs among that small minority who are the most sexually active (Anderson, 1989), a postulate we are already familiar with from the last chapter.

To state that the most sexually active are more influential in the spread of sexually transmitted diseases than the less sexually active is to lay oneself open to those old charges against social scientists of ponderous banality. But the argument is more than just a truism. Reports of the numbers of respondents' sexual partners in studies of men who have sex with men show heavily skewed distributions, with a small minority of the sample accounting for the majority of all reported partners. Thus the Project Sigma study, based on interviews in 1987–88 with a non-clinic sample of 930 men, showed that 42 per cent of the sample reported ten or fewer male partners in the previous five years, with a median figure of 16 partners, but 5 per cent of respondents reported 200 or more. The equivalent figures for 'penetrative partners' (that is, those with whom the respondent engaged in ano-genital sex) showed that 80 per cent reported ten or fewer male penetrative partners in the previous five years (with a median of three penetrative partners), but 4 per cent of respondents reported 50 or more (Davies et al., 1990: 105–106). The implication for epidemic spread is clear: while a substantial reduction in risk behaviour among the majority of gay men is a major health education achievement, it is the behaviour of the small minority reporting large numbers of partners which is the important determinant of epidemic spread – if they too are switching to safer sex, then a falling HIV incidence is assured.

Attempts have been made, in partner studies where one partner is HIV positive, to estimate the transmissibility of HIV through same-gender ano-genital intercourse. DeGruttola et al. (1989) estimated the risk of transmission at about 5 to 30 per thousand receptive anal exposures, but emphasised that there appeared to be great variation in infectivity (see also the section on heterosexual transmission, p. 43 below).

Variations in risk practices among men who have sex with men will be a topic for discussion in Chapter 4. What can be noted here are the variations within this transmission category in HIV prevalence. One of the largest cohorts of men who have sex with men is the Multicenter AIDS Cohort Study (MACS) being conducted in Baltimore/ Washington, Chicago, Pittsburgh and Los Angeles with a sample enrolment of 3,262 initially HIV-negative men. Like any cohort study concerned with this transmission category, reservations can be expressed about the representativeness of the sample, not least the clinic-based sample recruitment strategy (Kaslow et al., 1987), but the very size of the sample makes it useful for identifying socio-demographic differences in HIV-positivity, and for plotting changes over time. Although only 5 per cent of the cohort is non-white, rates of HIV positivity among Blacks were significantly greater in the Baltimore/Washington and Chicago samples in the period from 1984 to 1989. In Chicago, rates were also significantly higher for Hispanics (Kingsley et al., 1991). Few American epidemiological studies gather social class data so it is impossible to ascertain whether these and other data on higher HIV rates among non-whites simply reflect differences of wealth and status (an association noted earlier in African data) or whether they are an indication of the greater isolation and discrimination experienced by non-white gay men. The non-white segment of the MACS sample reported relatively higher frequencies of receptive anal intercourse and anal douching, more extensive histories of sexually transmitted diseases and a greater propensity to drug use and needle-sharing (Easterbrook et al., 1991).

Although the majority of newly reported cases of AIDS among gay men continue to be those of men in their thirties and forties, some cohort studies show that younger men are substantially more likely than older cohort members to become HIV positive. In the MACS study, men aged under 35 were at about one and a half times greater risk of seroconversion than those aged 35 and over (Easterbrook et al., 1991: 336). An English study of an opportunistic sample of gay men who had previously tested negative for HIV found an incidence rate for retested men aged over 44 of 1 per cent. But the comparable incidence rate for those aged under 25 was 6 per cent (Kaye and Miller, 1991). However, as we shall see in Chapter 4, there is some doubt about whether younger gay men are in fact experiencing more penetrative intercourse proportionately than their older peers.

Samples of men recruited in genito-urinary medicine clinics show significantly higher prevalences of HIV than samples recruited through other means such as gay organisations and the gay press. Project Sigma, a sample of the latter type, has reported on the HIV prevalence among that portion of their London sample who reported recent clinic attendance compared to the HIV prevalence among non-attenders, with prevalences of 16 per cent and 4 per cent respectively (Hunt et al., 1990).

Boulton and Weatherburn (1990), reviewing studies of bisexuality and HIV transmission, state that, in the developed world, HIV prevalence rates are in most countries significantly lower for bisexual men than for exclusively homosexual men. This is not true of some developing countries such as Mexico (see, for example, Izazola et al., 1991).

Data on 58 transsexuals in Sydney showed an HIV prevalence of 21 per cent (Alan et al., 1989), a prevalence rate that may well be higher than that found in Sydney gay men of a similar age. Three-quarters of these transsexuals were involved in prostitution. Studies of transvestites also show very high levels of HIV positivity – 69 per cent in Atlanta, Georgia (Elifson et al., 1990) and 56 per cent in Milan (Galli et al., 1990) – but these were exclusively prostitute transvestite populations.

The determination of HIV positivity among male prostitute populations is clearly a potentially important issue, in view of the earlier discussion of transmission dynamics and the potentially pivotal role of a small minority of very sexually active persons in epidemic spread. Of course, high prevalences of HIV do not necessarily indicate an involvement of male prostitution in epidemic spread, provided safer sex is being consistently practised. Risk behaviour data will be reported at length in Chapter 4 but, to anticipate a little, there is a small number of studies of male prostitution which report both high prevalences of HIV and high levels of risk behaviour. The Atlanta study of transvestite prostitutes reported above is a case in point, with 80 per cent of the 45 respondents reporting extensive receptive anal intercourse (Elifson et al., 1990). An earlier study of the non-transvestite male prostitute street population in Atlanta also revealed high levels of unsafe sex and an HIV prevalence of 25 per cent (Elifson et al., 1989). Similar levels of HIV were found in a small study of London male prostitutes (Tomlinson et al., 1991b). The largest study sample of male prostitutes is that of 211 respondents in Morse et al.'s (1991) New Orleans study; here the HIV prevalence rate was 17.5 per cent. Tabet et al.'s (1991) study indicated a still lower prevalence among male prostitutes in Albuquerque, New Mexico. These latter data are not entirely consistent with the earlier hypothesis of a pivotal role in epidemic spread for male prostitutes, suggesting instead that areas of low prevalence among gay men may also be areas of low HIV prevalence among male prostitutes, with male prostitutes possibly reflecting rather than influencing local prevalence rates. Transvestite prostitute populations, with their strong emphasis on receptive anal intercourse, may be untypical of wider male prostitute populations where anal intercourse may be a less common practice (see Chapter 4).

Another area of epidemiological uncertainty is to be found in debates around a possible 'second wave' of HIV infection among men who have sex with men. Some studies have indicated increases in new HIV cases in the late 1980s. In the aforementioned MACS study, for example, the Chicago cohort showed a fall in HIV incidence from 6.0 per cent in the last six months of 1984 to 0.0 per cent in the last six months of 1988. But in 1989, the Chicago incidence rate was 2.1 per cent for the first six months and 1.6 per cent for the last six months (Kingsley et al., 1991). However, the Chicago cohort was the only one of the four MACS centres to record an increase in incidence in 1989. Another study recording an end-of-decade increase in incidence is the Amsterdam gay men's cohort (van den Hoek et al., 1990). These findings, suggesting that a second wave of new infections may be occurring, are supported by reported upturns in rectal gonorrhoea infections among clinic samples of gay men in the USA (Handsfield, 1989) and the UK (Riley, 1991). Reports from Project Sigma also indicate an increase in the frequency of anal intercourse between 1988 and 1989: there were increases in the proportion of the sample engaging in anal intercourse in the previous year (Davies, 1989; Hunt et al., 1991). However, as will be seen in Chapter 4, such data must be interpreted cautiously: they may be indicative of a move towards what has been termed 'negotiated safety' – the practising of penetrative sex, but only with a regular partner deemed uninfected. If one considers the Project Sigma data on the mean number of penetrative sexual partners in the previous year, then a slight rise is evident (from 2.2 to 2.5 partners), but this is not a statistically significant change (Hunt et al., 1991).

At the start of the epidemic very little evidence was available on the prevalence of homosexual behaviour in the population. The only scientific data available on the extent of same-gender sexual contact were to be found in the 'Kinsey Report' from the 1940s (Kinsey et al., 1948). Indeed, there was a widespread feeling that scientific enquiry on sexual behaviour was an unwarranted intrusion into personal privacy, a feeling reportedly shared by Mrs Thatcher, whose government declined to fund the UK National Survey on Sexual Attitudes and Lifestyles (fortunately, a charitable trust, the Wellcome Foundation, picked up the tab).

Kinsey's data had indicated it was misleading to represent homosexual behaviour as clearly divided from heterosexual behaviour. Instead a continuum should be envisaged with just under 40 per cent of the male population having undergone, since adolescence, at least one same-gender sexual encounter involving orgasm. The same data indicated that 30 per cent of males had been actively homosexual for a period of at least three years between the ages of 16 and 55, and that 6 per cent of males were exclusively homosexual throughout their lives

(1948: 650–857). However, Kinsey's data were collected from volunteers; it was unclear whether similar results would be found among representative samples, and national surveys of sexual behaviour were commissioned in a number of countries.

A national survey had in fact been conducted in the USA in 1970 but the results went unpublished because of disputes between the investigators – the so-called 'long lost survey of sex' (Turner, 1989). When the results were finally published they showed a much lower prevalence of same-gender sexual activity than the Kinsey Report had indicated. The national data showed that 20 per cent of American men aged 21 or over had sexual contact to orgasm with another male at some time in their lives (the comparable figure in Kinsey was 40 per cent). Only 2 per cent reported such contact in the previous year, compared to Kinsey's figure of 6 per cent exclusively homosexual respondents (Fay et al., 1989). These data have themselves been the cause of controversy concerning possible reporting biases and one of the national survey authors comments that 'given the long history of discrimination and oppression of people who have same-gender sexual contacts, it is reasonable to expect that some men with such experience will conceal it in a survey' (Turner, 1989: S64). However, results of a number of surveys from different countries have now become available, with very similar results on the prevalence of same-gender sexual contacts. A Norwegian survey of 10,000 adults was the first to report. Their prevalence of men reporting same-gender contacts within the previous three years was 1.3 per cent (Sundet et al., 1988) and indirect indications of reporting biases (for example, rural–urban differences in reported prevalence) were noticeably absent (Sundet, personal communication). These Norwegian prevalence data were subsequently followed by comparable reports from Britain (the NATSSAL study) and France. British data showed 6.1 per cent of men reporting some kind of homosexual experience and 1.4 per cent reporting a male sexual partner within the last two years; while a response bias cannot be excluded, no evidence of any reporting bias was found (Wellings et al., 1994). A large French telephone survey reported that 4.1 per cent of the male respondents had at least one same-gender sexual contact in their lifetime and 1.1 per cent had a same-gender sexual contact in the past year (Analyse des Comportements Sexuels en France, 1992).

Injecting drug users (IDUs)

Drug injectors are thought to have first become infected with HIV in 1975 in New York, in 1978 in Italy (Moss, 1988) and in 1980 in Amsterdam (van Haastrecht et al., 1991).It is thought that around half all the cumulative cases of HIV infection in Europe are among injecting drug users; prevalences are uneven, with the heaviest concentrations occurring in Italy, Spain, southern France and Scotland. Prevalences are also uneven within countries: there are international differences in HIV prevalence between IDUs in different Italian cities (Tempesta and Di Giannantonio, 1990) and between different American cities. While the prevalence of HIV among IDUs in New York and New Jersey has been in excess of 40 per cent since at least the mid-1980s (Mamor et al., 1987; Weiss et al., 1985; Des Jarlais and Friedman, 1994), cities in the American Midwest like Dayton, Ohio, still have an HIV prevalence rate of less than 2 per cent among drug injectors (Siegal et al., 1991). However, the best known contrast in local prevalence rates is to be found in Scotland. In 1985 blood samples taken from IDUs in the Muirhouse district of Edinburgh were retrospectively tested for HIV: the findings, that half the sample were HIV positive (Robertson et al., 1986), created a sensation and led to media headlines like AIDS CITY. Subsequently, similar HIV prevalences were being reported in nearby Dundee. But forty miles down the motorway from Edinburgh lies Glasgow. Like Edinburgh, Glasgow experienced an explosion in injecting drug use in the working-class housing schemes in the early 1980s with an influx of cheap brown heroin from Pakistan. An estimate of the numbers of injecting drug users in Glasgow in 1989 indicated a figure of between 7,000 and 12,000 (between 1.1 per cent and 1.9 per cent of the city population aged 15 to 55: Frischer et al., 1991). Drug users and drug dealers move freely between the two cities and Glasgow and Edinburgh drug users are frequently thrown together in Scottish prisons and drug treatment agencies. Yet the prevalence of HIV among Glasgow IDUs was only 1.8 per cent in 1990, 1.2 per cent in 1991 and 1.0 per cent in 1992 (Taylor et al., 1994). The issue of local differences in HIV prevalence among IDUs is one to which we shall return in Chapter 4.

The near-independence of the epidemic among drug users from that among men who have sex with men has been recognised since the mid-1980s and is most clearly evidenced in the continuing low prevalence rate among IDUs in San Francisco. In a recent study of more than 3,000 methadone clinic attenders in the San Francisco Bay area, HIV rates for those male IDUs who had sex with men was 32.5 per cent, but HIV prevalence was only 8 per cent for the sample of IDUs as a whole (Reardon et al., 1991).

Other studies have also shown that, within a given locality, those IDUs who are infected show distinctive socio-demographic patterns. The IDU epidemic is, in fact, more internally differentiated than the gay epidemic. Most American studies, for example, show considerably higher prevalences among Black IDUs: in the San Francisco study, cited above, the HIV prevalence for African-Americans was 25 per cent, while for white IDUs it was 3 per cent. Other US studies (but not the San Francisco study) show higher prevalences among Hispanic IDUs. Gender differences are also apparent in rates of HIV positivity among drug injectors. In Glasgow, with an estimated ratio of male injectors to female injectors of 2.6 to one (Frischer et al., 1991), there appear to be slightly more HIV-positive female IDUs than males.

In a curious reversal of the situation found in epidemiological studies of men who have sex with men, which were discussed in the previous section, clinic samples of drug injectors have in the past shown *lower* prevalences of HIV than community samples; this was true of both the USA (Lampinen et al., 1992) and the UK (Haw et al., 1992). The clinic studies of gay men are drawn from genito-urinary medicine clinics and are thought to include disproportionate numbers of 'fast-lane' gay men with higher HIV rates. The clinic samples of drug injectors are drawn from drug treatment agencies and these samples too might be thought to show rather high HIV prevalences, since it is known that IDUs attending drug treatment programmes are older on average than those not in treatment (see, for example, Drucker and Vermund, 1989 on the New York methadone treatment programmes) and may therefore have been exposed to the risks of HIV infection for a longer period. Yet this assumption of a higher HIV prevalence rate in such clinic samples is often confounded. In a sample of 534 London IDUs where 22 per cent were recruited from 13 drug treatment agencies and the rest were recruited as a 'street' sample (using networks of IDUs known to the interviewers), 52 of the 63 HIV positives in the sample were found in the street sample (Haw et al., 1992). The overall HIV prevalence rate in this study of 12.8 per cent contrasts with a rate of 1.7 per cent reported in another London study recruiting drug injectors from eight of the city's drug treatment agencies (Public Health Laboratory Service, 1991).

The explanation for this epidemiological puzzle remains unclear. Of course, only a minority of IDUs are enrolled in drug treatment programmes: 35,000 of New York's estimated 200,000 IDUs were enrolled in methadone maintenance programmes in 1988 (Drucker and Vermund, 1989) and Frischer (1992) has calculated that a similar proportion of Glasgow's estimated 9,500 IDUs were in treatment in 1989. Those enrolled in treatment programmes may have been atypical in their risk exposure in such a way as to produce lower infection rates. A second possibility may be the reluctance of drug agency workers to enrol a client in testing studies where they already know or suspect the client to be HIV positive, with a consequent artefactual deflation of the study's HIV prevalence rate. Whatever the reasons, it may be that the scale of the HIV epidemic among IDUs has been under-reported, since most prevalence studies are based on clinic samples. The increasing practice of offering oral methadone to HIV-positive drug injectors attending treatment agencies may now be reversing this tendency for clinic samples of IDUs to report lower infection rates than community samples, attracting large numbers of HIV-positive injectors into treatment agencies.

The numbers of new cases of AIDS among IDUs continues to rise in most developed countries, reflecting the large increase in HIV infections in the early 1980s. But just as many local studies around 1987 found that the prevalence of HIV had stabilised among men who have sex with men (see above), so also there are now increasing numbers of reports of stabilisation of HIV prevalence among local populations of drug injectors. Des Jarlais and associates (1991) have reported the stabilisation of HIV prevalence among New York and Bangkok IDUs at 46 per cent and 34 per cent respectively. Glasgow's low and stable prevalence rate has already been reported. London studies indicate a stable or declining HIV prevalence of 8 per cent (Stimson, 1993).

The course of the IDU epidemic seems to have followed that of the gay men's epidemic with a three-year time-lag, with HIV prevalences among IDUs levelling out in many cities around 1990. These data need to be interpreted cautiously and are subject to quite wide confidence intervals. Table 3.2 indicates that, although the likelihood is that HIV prevalence among Glasgow IDUs remained stable between 1990 and 1992, it is nevertheless possible that prevalence increased in that period from 0.5 to 1.9 per cent! Clearly, the studies will need to be continued for several years before final conclusions can be drawn.

Reasons for this apparent stabilisation will be considered in more detail in Chapter 4. However, as was the case in studies of HIV among men who have sex with men, it seems likely that reductions in risk behaviour (in this case reductions in needle-sharing) have played a large part in limiting HIV spread.

However, local populations of HIV-positive injectors may vary for reasons that have nothing to do with changes in patterns of infection. This population change may stem from a number of causes. One factor is migration, although of course out-migration of HIV-positive drug injectors may be balanced by equivalent in-migration. Another factor

Table 3.2   *Prevalence of HIV among repeated community samples of Glasgow IDUs, 1990–92*

	no. tested	%age HIV+	95% Confidence interval
1990	454	1.8	0.5–3.0
1991	514	1.2	0.2–2.1
1992	484	1.0	0.1–1.9

Source: adapted from Taylor et al., 1994

is the mortality rate for HIV-positive IDUs: few of these deaths are directly AIDS-related, most of them being classed as overdoses or suicides (Galli et al., 1991; Frischer et al., 1993). Frischer and his colleagues' calculations of mortality among Glasgow IDUs indicate an all-cause mortality rate considerably in excess of UK Home Office estimates, suggesting that a degree of undercounting may be occurring. Finally, population attrition may also be caused by cessation of injecting: studies of HIV prevalence among samples of current injectors, whether recruited in drug treatment agencies or on the streets, will be unable to pick up HIV-positive ex-injectors. A pioneering pre-AIDS study attempted to trace a sample of heroin users recruited some ten years previously; a third of those who could be traced had ceased heroin use in the interim (Stimson and Oppenheimer, 1982). These sources of attrition in the drug-injecting population may lead to a paradoxical situation where a number of new cases of HIV infection may continue to occur each year among drug injectors but the HIV prevalence rate among IDUs remains constant: the annual incidence rate simply replaces that fraction of previous HIV-positive IDUs who are lost each year through attrition, be it differential out-migration, differential mortality, or differential cessation of injecting.

Attempts have been made to quantify the transmissibility of HIV through needle-sharing. Chin, in his Florence conference keynote address, cited WHO calculations of a transmission rate of between 3 and 10 transmissions per thousand exposures (Chin, 1991). Such calculations are of limited value, however, since the term 'needle-sharing' actually refers to a range of quite different activities with very different likelihoods of transmission: sharing a single 'hit' dissolved in blood drawn up into the syringe may represent a different order of risk to the re-use of previously discarded and rinsed injecting equipment. Some further indication of transmissibility is given by calculation of infection rates due to needle-stick injuries, although here too the degree of exposure may vary considerably. Gill et al.(1991) have summarised the published literature on occupational needle-stick injuries. The most comprehensive study is that of surveillance by the US Centers for Disease Control (Atlanta) of the results of all occupational needle-stick injuries reported to Atlanta. Out of 1,127 percutaneous (skin-penetrating) exposures up to 1990 only 4 resulted in HIV transmission (Tokars et al., 1990), a transmission rate comparable with the WHO estimate.

The prevalence of injecting drug use itself is a further area of epidemiological uncertainty. In the UK general practitioners and others are required to notify the Home Office of the names of all drug injectors but this requirement is not always followed (in the USA a similar scheme of reporting to the Narcotics Registry is also incomplete). It is recognised that the Notifications Scheme substantially undercounts drug injectors, particularly in certain cities. Glasgow, the city with probably the largest UK population of drug injectors outside London, had only 142 notifications of injectors in 1989, but an estimated IDU population of 9,400 (Frischer et al., 1991). National surveys, such as the UK's National Sexual Attitudes and Lifestyles Survey, have enquired about injecting drug use, as have some large-scale surveys of young people's health and behaviour (for example Ford, 1991). Fears of sampling bias and under-reporting in such surveys have led some researchers to investigate alternative methods of estimating the size of the drug-injecting population.

One such alternative method is the 'mark/recapture' approach which has long been used by field ecologists to estimate the size of wild animal populations. The method involves tagging a group of captured deer, for example, releasing them and then capturing and examining a second group of deer to see what proportion of the second population are 'recaptures', tagged on the earlier occasion; the size of the overall deer population is derived from the proportion of such recaptures. Applying the method to estimating the size of populations such as drug injectors typically involves comparing two partial populations of injectors, for example police arrest data and drug treatment agency data, and discovering the proportion of overlaps ('recaptures') between them. Confidentiality may be maintained by using a system of unnamed identifiers, such as date of birth, initial, and first part of postcode and by systems of 'third party' record linkage. The approach is discussed in detail by Hartnoll et al. (1985). The best known application of the mark/recapture technique is Drucker and Vermund's (1989) estimation of the population and demographic characteristics of Bronx injectors.

The use of a log linear model (Cormack, 1989; Frischer et al., 1991) represents a further development of the technique. The comparison of overlaps between two partial populations necessitates the (perhaps unrealistic) assumption that the two source populations are independent from each other – no cross-referral, for example, between drug treatment agencies and the police. However, Frischer's estimation of the Glasgow injector population involved the collation of unnamed identifier data from a wide variety of sources (police arrest data, Home Office notifications, the Scottish HIV Test Register, drug rehabilitation centres, community drug projects, syringe-exchanges and hospital data) and was able to waive the independence requirement – in fact, modelling proceeds by reference to the degree of dependence between different sources.

The remaining uncertainties concerning the mark/recapture technique centre on the issue of sample heterogeneity – the different propensity of some injectors to appear in some of the partial populations used in the prevalence calculation. Clearly local populations of drug injectors are highly heterogeneous and this can, in principle, pose considerable problems for mark/recapture estimates. Cormack and others are continuing to explore possible mathematical solutions to the problem of sample heterogeneity in mark/recapture studies. A national mark/recapture study of the drug-injecting population is currently under way in Wales.

Haemophiliacs and transfusion recipients

The disastrous consequences are well known of the delays in protecting transfusion recipients and haemophiliacs from HIV infection. In the UK, the government has compensated sufferers and their families. In France, the former director of the Centre National de Transfusion Sanguine was charged with having offered for sale blood products he knew to be tainted and toxic, and the former director-general for health and the former director of the National Laboratory were charged with failure to assist endangered individuals.

In France and the UK approximately a third of all haemophiliacs are thought to be infected (AIDS Group of the UK Haemophilia Centres, 1989; *AIDS Letter*, 1992a). Those most likely to be infected are those whose clotting defect is most severe and who therefore had most recourse to Factor VIII, the clotting agent that (because it was extracted from large volumes of blood derived from many different donors) was frequently contaminated with HIV.

Ninety-four cases of AIDS as a result of blood transfusions had been reported in the UK up to December 1993. However, just over half of these patients had received their contaminated transfusions abroad, where contamination of blood supplies was frequently more common and where some countries at first lacked the resources to screen their blood supplies for HIV. Testing for antibodies to HIV-1 was introduced for UK blood donations in October 1985 (testing for antibodies to HIV-2 was introduced in June 1990). Newly infected donors cannot always be detected since antibodies to HIV may take up to three months to develop. However, it is thought that only one further case of HIV transmission by blood transfusion has occurred in the UK since screening was introduced; up to the end of March 1991 nearly 15 million UK blood donations had been screened for HIV (*AIDS Letter*, 1992b).

The belated protection of blood supplies and blood products did not have any impact on the numbers of AIDS cases until the late 1980s; the incidence of reported AIDS cases among haemophiliacs and transfusion recipients continued to rise steeply in the 1980s, as more and more pre-screening cases of HIV transmission came to light following their development of AIDS-related symptoms. New AIDS cases continue to be reported; in the year up 30 June 1994 in the USA 911 new cases were reported among haemophiliacs and 1,129 new cases were reported among transfusion recipients (reported by Centers for Disease Control and Prevention).

Heterosexual transmission

The disclosure in 1991 by Magic Johnson, the American sportsman, that he had contracted HIV by heterosexual transmission stimulated world-wide media interest almost on a par with Rock Hudson's terminal illness several years earlier. Magic Johnson's disclosure was the occasion for a press release from the World Health Organisation. Michael Merson, the replacement for Jonathan Mann as director of WHO's Global Programme on AIDS, was quoted as saying:

> The forthright revelation by Magic Johnson that he is infected with HIV drives home a basic truth about the AIDS pandemic. Mr Johnson is telling sexually active people that, whatever their sexual preference, they simply cannot afford to consider themselves invulnerable. You may choose to take the risk and have unprotected intercourse with a casual partner, but it may turn out to be a fatal error.

WHO went on to cite a range of figures on heterosexual spread. Three-quarters of the estimated 8–10 million adults with HIV have become infected by heterosexual transmission. Although very few of the early AIDS cases in the developed world were due to heterosexual transmission, many developed countries are now reporting an explosion in the numbers of such cases. It was estimated in 1991 that 100,000 adults in the USA had been infected heterosexually; there were 21,873 reported US AIDS cases infected by heterosexual transmission up to 30 June 1993.

The WHO press release was issued on Armistice Day but was part of a propaganda war. In the UK, for example, some (but not all) sections of the tabloid press have run a series of sceptical stories, editorials and features on the risks of heterosexual transmission (see Beharrell, 1992 for an extended analysis of UK press coverage on this topic). The low numbers of reported AIDS cases due to heterosexual transmission have been turned against the government view and used to argue against there being any danger to the heterosexual population. Researchers and gay activists have also been accused of constructing a false picture for their own ends of a burgeoning heterosexual epidemic.

The available statistics have been selectively cited to promote sharply differing viewpoints. We must pick our way through them with care. First off, it is true that very few reported UK AIDS cases to date are the result of heterosexual transmission – 861 cases out of 8,529 reported up to 31 December 1993. And it is also the case that the great majority of those heterosexual transmission cases occurred abroad (738 cases out of 861). However, the average latency period from infection with HIV to developing AIDS is at least seven years and probably longer (Anderson and Medley, 1988). And it is widely believed, because of more limited transmissibility (see pp. 48–51) and low rates of partner change, that the anticipated heterosexual HIV epidemic will build up more slowly than the epidemic among men who have sex with men (Johnson, 1988). Thus it is clear that the debate about a heterosexual epidemic should be conducted with reference to data on HIV cases rather than AIDS cases.

Table 3.3 draws on data from the UK government official HIV reporting schemes. It confirms that local heterosexual transmission is occurring, but the numbers still appear relatively small. Only a sixth (3,181) of all the 21,101 reported HIV cases were thought to involve heterosexual transmission and, of these, the clear majority involved infection abroad (largely in Africa, largely to African nationals). Of the remainder where details were known (662), two-thirds (430) were cases of 'secondary transmission' – men and women who had sex with injecting drug users or infected haemophiliacs, or infected blood transfusion recipients, or women who had sex with bisexual men. This left just 232 cases out of 21,101 reported where transmission appeared to have occurred as a result of a UK general heterosexual epidemic on similar lines to that found in Pattern II countries.

However, there are various reasons for supposing that official HIV reporting schemes in the UK and in other developed countries may be understating the extent of the heterosexual epidemic. One reason is that HIV-positive sexual partners of injecting drug users who are themselves injecting drug users are always assumed by the authorities to become infected by needle-sharing, although some at least may have

Table 3.3   *Heterosexual transmission of HIV-1 – UK case reports to 31 December 1993*

Gender:	Male	Female	Unknown	Total
Sexual transmission between men and women				
– 'high risk' partner	70	360	–	430
– other partner, abroad	1,232	1,056	8	2,296
– other partner, UK	81	151	–	232
– under investigation	99	124	–	223
All heterosexual transmission cases	1,482	1,691	8	3,181
All HIV cases	18,257	2,791	53	21,101

Source: Public Health Laboratory Service, 1994

become infected through unprotected intercourse (Bloor et al., 1991b). A second (and more important) reason lies in the differential propensity for different individuals to seek HIV testing. Infected persons who do not perceive themselves to have been at much risk of infection are unlikely to present themselves for voluntary HIV testing and will not appear in the HIV reporting scheme data. This is particularly likely where the infected person's only risk behaviour was unprotected heterosexual intercourse. The Cox Report in 1988 (Chief Medical Officer, 1988) estimated that only 10 per cent of those in the UK who were heterosexually infected at that time had been tested, compared to 50 per cent of those infected through homosexual contact. The differential propensity to seek testing is reinforced by the social pressures on some individuals to undergo testing: drug injectors seeking treatment in outpatient clinics, drug treatment agencies, dental surgeries and elsewhere have sometimes found themselves denied treatment unless they submit to testing.

Participation biases like those above have increasingly led epidemiologists to favour 'unlinked' anonymous HIV testing studies. In these, HIV prevalence is ascertained in treatment agency populations where the reason for attending the agency is unconnected with possible HIV transmission. Samples of blood or urine which are routinely taken for other laboratory tests are also tested for HIV, unless the patient spontaneously objects (Gill et al., 1989). In England and Wales in 1990, for example, 8,996 genito-urinary medicine clinic attenders were tested in this way and 69,091 pregnant women. Women attending London GUM clinics who were not known to have injected drugs had an HIV-1 prevalence of 0.2 per cent; a similar percentage of women receiving antenatal care in inner London also tested HIV positive. Elsewhere in England and Wales very few infected women were found in either GUM clinics or antenatal clinics (Public Health Laboratory Service, 1991). A parallel Scottish study of GUM clinic attenders in Edinburgh and Glasgow found a similar prevalence figure of 0.2 per cent among women not known to have injected drugs; among heterosexual males HIV prevalence was 0.4 per cent (Goldberg, personal communication). And a Scottish voluntary testing study of antenatal clinic attenders with 91 per cent participation showed an HIV prevalence rate among Edinburgh expectant mothers of 0.02 per cent (Goldberg et al., 1992) *after* self-reported IDUs and partners of IDUs had been excluded. Among blood donors donating blood for the first time 79 out of 1.9 million donations have proved positive, a prevalence rate of 0.004 per cent (*AIDS Letter*, 1992b), but potential donors who believe themselves to have been at risk of HIV infection are asked to self-defer.

Based on the unlinked anonymous HIV prevalence monitoring programme, a PHLS Working Group (the 'revised Day Report') has estimated the numbers of HIV-positive persons in England and Wales infected through heterosexual exposure up to the end of 1991 to be 6,500 (PHLS Working Group, 1993).

The unlinked testing programmes will continue and there should be no tabloid-style rush to judgement on the *future* course of the heterosexual epidemic. Clearly, the epidemic to date has not followed the African pattern; instead, the heterosexual epidemic in the developed world has been an epidemic of 'secondary transmission'. But this is not to say that a 'Pattern II' generalised heterosexual epidemic might not emerge in the future. The difficulty in making a definite forecast here lies in the probable slow-building nature of such a future epidemic, which makes its initial stages extremely difficult to detect epidemiologically.

The speed of epidemic spread of a sexually transmitted disease is the 'basic reproductive rate' – the average number of new infections produced by one infected subject. An infection will spread only if this variable exceeds 1.0. Anderson and May (1988) have estimated that the basic reproductive rate for the heterosexual community will actually be around that figure of 1.0. If it is less than 1.0, then some secondary transmission will continue to occur, but not widespread dissemination. If it is slightly more than 1.0, then dissemination will be so slow as to be virtually undetectable in the first stages of the epidemic when prevalence remains at low levels (Skegg, 1989). A basic reproductive rate of 1.1 would produce a doubling time of eight to fourteen years (compared to one to two years in some African countries). Thus, HIV prevalence in a general population sample might only rise from 0.1 per cent to 0.2 per cent over a ten-year period but still produce catastrophic prevalence levels in the twenty-first century. Such small changes in prevalence cannot be measured with statistical exactitude. The jury is still out.

If the future pattern of the heterosexual epidemic remains unclear, the current pattern is not. The UK pattern, reflected in Table 3.1, is found in a number of developed countries and contains a number of distinct components. Firstly, there is the component of HIV/AIDS cases among nationals from Pattern II countries. This component is strongest in those countries with a colonial legacy such as Britain, Belgium, Portugal and France; in the USA, almost a quarter of the 10,000 adult AIDS cases involving heterosexual contact reported up to July 1991 were persons born in Pattern II countries. The numbers of both HIV and AIDS cases among Pattern II nationals resident in the developed world are rising as a natural correlate of the continuing epidemic in their countries of origin. It is as well to be clear that the above data refer to the heterosexual AIDS epidemic. If all AIDS cases are considered, then a different picture emerges. In the EU countries for example, with the exception of Belgium, the majority of AIDS cases among foreigners are cases of other EU nationals or Americans (Haour-Knipe, 1991).

A second component of the heterosexual epidemic is that of the sexual partners of Pattern II nationals. This is a small component in most countries (only 1.5 per cent of the 10,000 American heterosexual transmission AIDS cases) but is represented as a large component in xenophobic discourses advocating travel restrictions and condoning discrimination and victimisation of African students and others. Ironically, it is possible that transmissions involving persons from Pattern II countries domiciled in the developed world may be counterbalanced by transmission by travellers from the developed world (sex tourists, holiday-makers, and migrant workers) to local sexual partners while visiting Third World countries. James Chin, the WHO's chief AIDS epidemiologist, has issued a warning about the possible epidemiological role of the sex tourist (Chin, 1988). Sex tourism infects local prostitute populations, leading to further epidemic spread locally and among other sex tourists. The recent rapid increases in HIV prevalence among prostitutes in favoured sex tourism destinations such as Bangkok (see Chapter 2) are likely to result in a future increase in developed world heterosexual infections. In respect of returning migrant workers, the South Korean experience is instructive. South Korea has very low levels of HIV infection but exactly half (n = 50) of all known HIV cases have been found among Korean nationals returning from overseas job assignments (Choi et al., 1991). A study of HIV among Dutch expatriates returning from Africa found an HIV prevalence of 0.4 per cent among the males and 0.1 per cent among the females (Houweling and Coutinho, 1991b).

A third component of the heterosexual epidemic is that of the sexual partners of infected haemophiliacs and infected transfusion recipients. This too is a small component. Centers for Disease Control (CDC) data on US women with AIDS showed that 4.1 per cent had become heterosexually infected from a blood product recipient (Berkelman et al., 1991). It is likely that the incidence of HIV cases among sexual partners of blood product recipients has already peaked: the US Multicenter Study of AIDS in Haemophilia reports no new cases of HIV among 135 female sexual partners of haemophiliacs between 1987 and 1989 (Killinger et al., 1990).

The same CDC data on US women with AIDS shows that the fourth component of the heterosexual epidemic, sex with bisexual men, is a shrinking component. In 1983–84, 21 per cent of women with AIDS were partners of bisexuals; in 1989–90 it was only 9 per cent (Berkelman et al., 1991). The limited overlap between the heterosexual epidemic and the epidemic among men who have sex with men was noted early on – witness the small number of infected women in San Francisco (Chaisson et al., 1987). This is despite the fact that several community samples of men who have sex with men indicate that around 5 per cent have a current female partner and about 10–15 per cent report at least one female partner in the previous year (Boulton and Weatherburn, 1990).

In many countries (the USA, Scotland, most of Southern Europe) the greatest component of heterosexual transmission cases is that of the sexual partners of injecting drug users. Moss, in an early review of HIV/AIDS infection among IDUs, called the epidemic among drug injectors 'the real heterosexual epidemic' (Moss, 1987), because of the potential for heterosexual spread of HIV to the sexual partners of drug injectors. In New York, probably the city in the developed world with the highest prevalence of HIV, 88 per cent of female AIDS cases due to heterosexual transmission reported sex with an IDU partner (Stoneburner et al., 1990). In Edinburgh, where the prevalence of HIV among IDUs has stabilised and where reported levels of needle-sharing have fallen, it is thought that heterosexual transmission is probably a more common cause of new infections among drug injectors than is needle-sharing (Ronald et al., 1992), signalling the possible local transformation of HIV from an epidemic to an endemic disease.

The importance of injecting drug use in secondary transmission may, in part, reflect the greater transmissibility of HIV between IDUs and their sexual partners. Padian (1990) has suggested in her review that there may be such differences in transmissibility. However, one reason for the pivotal role of IDUs in secondary transmission is simply the greater size of the heterosexually active IDU population relative to the size of the bisexually active population and the heterosexually active haemophiliac population. In New York alone the estimated IDU population is 200,000 (Drucker and Vermund, 1989).

The issue of differential transmissibility has already been touched on in Chapter 1. Although the average chance of infection may be only one or two in a thousand sexual acts, transmissibility may vary considerably under the influence of a number of different factors. This remains an issue around which there are considerable uncertainties (see the reviews by Johnson and Laga, 1990, Padian, 1990, and Skegg, 1989; see also data reported by de Vincenzi, 1994).

It appears that there are genetic differences in susceptibility to HIV infection (see, for example, Louie et al., 1991), but there is no evidence to link these genetic differences to other data showing increased transmissibility among American Blacks and Hispanics relative to whites (Padian, 1990). It may be that these apparent ethnic differences in transmissibility are epiphenomena masking an association of increased transmissibility with poverty. It also appears that transmissibility may vary between different strains of the virus. Like other viruses (most prominently the influenza viruses), HIV is subject to considerable variation. A number of molecular epidemiology projects are now in train exploring the possibility that some strains are more readily transmitted than others. As was noted in Chapter 2, it is already apparent that HIV-2 is less readily transmitted than HIV-1.

More certain than these supposed differences in transmissibility associated with viral strain, genetic differences and secondary transmission category, are those differences associated with gender, mode of intercourse, disease progression and the presence of other sexually transmitted diseases. It was originally thought that there was a rough parity between male and female infections in African countries, but there is now increasing evidence that more African women are infected than men (Chin, 1990). This disparity also seems to be true of Pattern I countries. The strongest suggestions of a gender difference are to be found in the New York data. Although New York has the greatest concentration of HIV-positive female drug injectors in the world, very few local reported AIDS cases have been ascribed to female-to-male heterosexual transmission. Of the 630 AIDS cases involving heterosexual transmission reported up to September 1989, 623 were female and just 7 were male (Stoneburner et al., 1990).

American and European studies of transmissibility between discordant couples (where one partner is initially positive and one is initially negative) all show greater rates of transmission from male to female than from female to male (see the review by Johnson and Laga, 1990). However, the numbers of cases involved (particularly in female-to-male transmission studies) have been small and it has been difficult to calculate precise differences in transmission rates. An EU study, co-ordinated at the European Centre for the Epidemiological Monitoring of AIDS in Paris, has collected data on 563 discordant heterosexual couples across the European Community. The mean probability of male-to-female transmission per sexual act was found to be 1.9 times (confidence interval 1.1 times to 3.3 times) that of female-to-male transmission (European Study Group on Heterosexual Transmission of HIV, 1992); in univariate analysis however, male/female differences in transmissibility did not reach statistical significance, possibly because of the small numbers of new infections recorded over the three-year study period (de Vincenzi, 1994). The hypothesis of male/female differences in transmissibility is consistent with gendered differences in transmission risk in respect of other sexually transmitted diseases such as gonorrhoea.

Transmissibility also seems to vary according to the types of sexual practice undertaken. The association of increased transmissibility with anal intercourse is well known. It has been estimated that heterosexual anal intercourse more than doubles the risk of male-to-female transmission (Padian et al., 1987). Intercourse during menses has been suggested as significantly increasing the risk of female-to-male transmission, although no supportive evidence for this was found in the above EU study (de Vincenzi, 1994). It may also be anticipated that any sexual activity that increases the likelihood of vaginal genital trauma will also increase the transmission risk. As an indication of the degree of epidemiological uncertainty that still surrounds the issue of transmissibility, it should be emphasised that most of the discordant couples studies reviewed by Johnson and Laga (1990) were unable to demonstrate any relationship between risk of transmission on the one hand and the length of the couple's sexual relationship, or the number of their sexual contacts, on the other.

Another influence on transmissibility is that of disease progression in the index case (infected party). As individuals progress towards AIDS their infectivity appears to increase, possibly because of an associated increase in levels of infectious virus in semen and cervical secretions. In a study of twenty-four female partners of infected haemophiliacs, three women became infected more than four years after their partner's initial infection, coinciding with a fall in T-helper lymphocyte counts (indicating a fall in white blood cells) in their partners (Goedert et al., 1987). This suggests that, in the absence of a switch to increased condom use, levels of partner infection will rise as more and more index cases develop AIDS. An early study of rates of heterosexual transmission among the partners of a large sample of haemophiliacs indicated a transmission rate of only 10 per cent (Centers for Disease Control, 1987). In contrast, a four-year follow-up of ninety Italian couples recently reported a transmission rate of 48 per cent (Falciano et al., 1991). In the EU Discordant Couples Study the rate of transmission was five per thousand exposures (95 per cent confidence interval, 1.4 to 13.1) when the index case (initially infected partner) was at an advanced stage of the disease, but the transmission rate was only 0.7 per thousand (95 per cent confidence interval, 0.3 to 1.4) when the index case was pre-symptomatic (de Vincenzi, 1994).

If infectiousness is associated with 'viral load' (levels of infectious virus in bodily fluids) then infectiousness may also be expected to be greater at the point when the index case is first infected, because of the initial absence of antibodies. This initial, pre-antibodies heightened infectiousness may help explain the seemingly characteristic epidemic pattern in some populations (notably drug injector populations), namely the pattern of sudden explosive epidemic spread followed by near-stabilisation of prevalence. However, there is no certain epidemiological evidence bearing on this hypothesised greater infectiousness prior to antibody development.

The area of greatest scientific controversy in respect of transmission studies is that of the search for 'co-factors' – co-infections which may facilitate HIV transmission. Various candidate co-factors have been proposed, such as cytomegalovirus (CMV) and Epstein–Barr virus (EBV), but the strongest epidemiological evidence centres on a co-factorial role for several other sexually transmitted diseases – most notably chancroid, syphilis and herpes simplex infection. Early evidence of an association between HIV and other STDs was difficult to interpret because it was recognised that a history of STDs could merely be a 'marker' for rapid partner change and that it was the latter factor that was causally associated with HIV positivity. Nevertheless, a theoretical case could be made out for a co-factorial role because other STD infections could increase a person's susceptibility to HIV infection through their impact on the immune system.

To the above theoretical case for an increased *susceptibility* to HIV among persons with other STDs, must now be added epidemiological evidence of an increased *infectivity* among persons with other STDs. A series of important studies of Nairobi prostitutes and their male clients by Plummer and his associates has shown that other STDs greatly increase the likelihood of HIV transmission because of concomitant genital ulceration facilitating viral exit and entry (see the overview by Cameron, 1990). Those male clients who developed genital ulcer disease following prostitute contact were significantly more likely to become HIV positive, suggesting that genital ulcer disease in the women enhanced transmission. It was estimated that the transmission rate after a single exposure to a woman in the Nairobi prostitute study (more than 80 per cent of whom were HIV positive) was not 1 per 1,000 (as in the EC study) but 80 per 1,000 (Cameron et al., 1988). These findings may also explain the association found in some studies between transmission and non-circumcision, since genital ulcerations are frequently found on the foreskin. Chancroid is the STD most strongly associated with genital ulceration. Thirty-three per cent of the Nairobi prostitute cohort had chancroid infections (Cameron, 1990). Chancroid is uncommon in developed countries, although a study of genito-urinary medicine clinic attenders in New York found an association between male chancroid infection and female-to-male HIV transmission (Telzak et al., 1991). Syphilis and herpes simplex infection may also produce genital ulceration. Enhanced transmisability was also associated with genital infections in the EU Discordant Couples Study; most of the infections reported in this study were cases of herpes or candida (de Vincenzi, 1994).

The Nairobi findings touch upon a second controversial issue, namely the role of prostitution in heterosexual transmission. Male prostitution was discussed in an earlier section and Chapter 2 illustrated the important role of female prostitution in the African epidemic as an epidemiological 'core group'. However, it is by no means clear that female prostitution is playing an equivalent role in heterosexual transmission in the developed world. Tabloids and 'quality' papers alike have carried sensational reports of prostitutes 'infecting' clients on a large scale (for example, the uncritical reports in the *Scotsman* and the *Independent* on 14 December 1991 of Paris police claims that prostitutes in the Bois de Boulogne were infecting up to 40 clients a day and had already 'contaminated' up to 14,000 clients!). Ironically and in contrast, it seems likely that it is the behaviour of prostitute women that is one of the main bulwarks against an African-style heterosexual epidemic in the developed world.

Studies of HIV prevalence among prostitute women in developed countries have shown considerable local variability. Preliminary results of the CDC collaborative multi-centre study in the USA (Campbell, 1990) showed HIV prevalences varying between 0.0 per cent (Las Vegas) and 55 per cent (Newark/Jersey City). Similar variations in HIV prevalences have been found between different European cities. These local variations are a consequence of the overlap between injecting drug use and female prostitution. Those cities with the highest HIV prevalence rates among prostitute women are also the cities with high HIV prevalence rates among IDUs. This is clearest in Southern Europe: a prevalence study of over 300 prostitute women in four Italian centres found an HIV prevalence rate of 36 per cent among drug-injecting prostitutes but only 1.6 per cent among the non-injectors (Tirelli et al., 1989); in Oviedo, in Spain, a study of over 500 prostitute women found an HIV prevalence of 48 per cent among IDUs, but only 7 per cent among non-injectors (Palacio et al., 1989). In Glasgow, where more than 70 per cent of female street prostitutes are IDUs, the prevalence of HIV in a sample of over 200 such women was only 2.5 per cent (confidence interval: 0.7 to 6.3) (McKeganey et al., 1992), a prevalence rate equivalent to that found among community samples of Glasgow IDUs (Haw et al., 1992): where rates of infection among IDUs are low, then rates of infection among drug-injecting prostitute women will also be low.

Day's wide-ranging review (1988) suggests another possible link between injecting drug use and HIV prevalence among prostitute women: some non-injecting women may have been infected by their drug-injecting boyfriends. Many prostitute women who are accustomed to use condoms with commercial partners seek to distinguish the intimacy of private sexual relationships by not using condoms (Day et al., 1988; Barnard, 1992).

The size of the client population for prostitute women is difficult to calculate, for obvious reasons. A Swiss national telephone survey has provided estimates of commercial sex contacts both in Switzerland and abroad: 12 per cent (95 per cent confidence interval: 10 per cent to 14 per cent) of Swiss males aged 17–30 reported previous sexual experience with prostitutes; 1.2 per cent of Swiss males aged 17–45 had paid for sex abroad in the previous year (Hausser et al., 1991). In the UK's NATSSAL study only 1.8 per cent of males reported paying for sex with a woman in the past five years (Johnson et al., 1994).

Conclusion

There is a story about a statistician awakened in his bedroom by a psychopathic intruder: asked whether he preferred to die by stabbing or strangulation, the statistician said he needed more data before he could decide. A refusal to rush to judgement may be a strategy of self-defence as well as sound professional practice and some informed judgements need to be made now about the current course of the HIV epidemic in the developed world. Nevertheless, in at least one important area (the course of the heterosexual epidemic), some things remain too close to call.

However, even in respect of the heterosexual epidemic, some firm conclusions can also be drawn. In the first place, the numbers of heterosexually transmitted AIDS cases in the developed world will continue to increase in the medium term. There is no short-term prospect of this category of cases peaking because there is no evidence of a current peaking of heterosexually transmitted HIV cases and because the epidemiological pattern of AIDS cases represents that of HIV cases seven or so years previously.

Secondly, a continuing increase (at least in the short term) seems likely in heterosexually transmitted HIV cases in the developed world. This increase will have at least three components. There will be an increase in the numbers of HIV-positive persons from Pattern II countries resident in Pattern I countries: if HIV prevalence continues to rise in developing countries, this will be reflected in a rise in prevalence amongst persons from those countries domiciled in the developed world. There will also be a rise in the numbers of nationals from Pattern I countries who become HIV positive while abroad (recall the returning Dutch ex-patriates and recall the German sex tourists interviewed in Bangkok). And it is also likely that the numbers of 'secondary' heterosexual transmissions will also show an increase, at least in the short term. The sexual partners of HIV-positive drug injectors may become increasingly at risk as their positive partners' infectiousness increases, a consequence of their progression to ARC/AIDS: if experience in Italy (where HIV infection spread relatively early in the epidemic among drug injectors) is any guide, then around half of the regular sexual partners of HIV-positive injectors may eventually become HIV positive themselves (Falciano et al., 1991).

Beyond these likely increases, what remains too close to call is the possibility in developed countries of a slow-building (but eventually devastating) *general* (as opposed to secondary) heterosexual epidemic. Such epidemics are impossible to detect statistically in their early stages. However, there are three reasons for cautious optimism: firstly, transmissibility rates appear much lower in the developed world than in Africa because of the much lower prevalences of other sexually transmitted diseases which cause genital ulceration; secondly, prostitute women, who formed an epidemiological 'core group' in the African epidemic, continue to show low HIV prevalences (except among drug-injecting prostitutes) and widely practise safer commercial sex (see Chapter 4); and, thirdly, some mathematical models based on estimated transmissibility rates and on survey reports of partner change indicate that a general heterosexual epidemic is unlikely to be self-sustaining. Thus, the data from the Norwegian population survey reported above have been used to indicate that the heterosexual HIV epidemic could not be sustained in Norway if the transmissibility rate is below one in a hundred sexual acts and no new infection is imported from outside this population (Stigum et al., 1989); the transmission rate studies reported earlier do indeed indicate a rate below this one in a hundred ratio.

General heterosexual epidemic or not, it is clear that in the medium term cases of heterosexual transmission will remain a minority of all HIV-positive cases in the developed world. The revised Day Report estimated there were 13,900 HIV-positive men who have sex with men and 2,000 HIV-positive drug injectors in England and Wales at the end of 1991 (PHLS Working Group, 1993). Most positive cases will continue to be found among men who have sex with men and among injecting drug users. The rapid transmission rates of the early 1980s are a thing of the past and in both transmission categories it appears that HIV prevalences are now near-stable. But near-stable prevalence rates does not mean that there will be no new cases, because of the phenomenon of population attrition. Rather, constant HIV prevalence in a study group cohort implies continuing numbers of new cases to replace earlier HIV cases that disappear from the study.

4

Sociological Studies of Risk Behaviour

For purposes of exposition, a distinction has been made hitherto between epidemiological and sociological studies of the HIV epidemic, but the untenability of the distinction was already apparent in previous chapters, where the narrative strayed repeatedly beyond the reporting of the unfolding pattern of the epidemic – strayed into reports of behavioural change (reductions in the numbers of penetrative sexual partners among men who have sex with men), into references to the rich erotic culture of Brazil, and into the association of Third World prostitution with those economic forces creating an extensive migrant male labour force.

Abandoning the previous epidemiological–sociological distinction allows us to subject some of the assumptions of epidemiological reports to critical scrutiny. In particular, the assumption may be questioned that epidemiological findings are scientifically neutral, objective facts. The classification of epidemiological case reports into different exposure categories ('sexual intercourse between men', 'injecting drug use', etc.) can serve as an illustrative example. To classify cases by reported exposure category is simultaneously to represent the epidemic in a particular form and few social representations have a more privileged status in our culture than official statistics. The adoption of particular classificatory schemes guides our seeing: the UK epidemic is represented selectively as concentrated, for example, among men who have sex with men, or among Londoners, depending on the choice of tabular classification.

Such selective representation has, of course, a high degree of pragmatic utility in representing disease epidemiology, but any pragmatic scheme of representation also carries certain dangers. Most importantly, these schemes have a self-fulfilling character. The ways of seeing that are endorsed by the adoption of particular classificatory schemes become themselves the basis for the everyday interpretative acts of those who compile and construct the statistical tables. Faced with case reports of HIV-positive persons who report, for example, both heterosexual intercourse and syringe-sharing, those who operate the official reporting schemes must choose between competing classifications in decisions on case allocation (Bloor et al., 1991b). Small wonder if the choice is made on the basis of prior knowledge of which have been the most common exposure categories, a prior knowledge that is itself predicated on the earlier case-allocation decisions that were the building blocks of the earlier exposure-category statistics. Epidemiological taxonomies may be factitious rather than strictly factual.

Gephart (1988) has used the term 'ethnostatistics' to describe the study of statistical case-allocation and compilation decisions. Shilts (1987) reports that, in the early days of the American epidemic, physicians reporting cases to the Atlanta Centers for Disease Control disbelieved drug-injecting AIDS sufferers who denied any homosexual involvements: ethnostatistical decisions were based on prior representations of the epidemic as a 'gay plague'. All social representations are bases for social actions, social actions which may serve to confirm and reinforce those earlier social representations.

This is not to claim that HIV/AIDS statistics are fictitious as well as factitious; after all needle-sharing did eventually receive due epidemiological recognition as a transmission route. Rather it is to claim that statistical representations of the epidemic are not neutral representations: they are sets of discursive practices of particular power because of their perceived objective and scientific character. They shape our understandings of the epidemic and are linked with other popular discourses of the epidemic from the liberal to the homophobic and xenophobic.

For good or ill, therefore, most sociological studies of risk behaviour have centred on particular epidemiological exposure categories. And, for good or ill, those studies are reported here according to similar categorical sub-divisions – risk behaviour among men who have sex with men, among injecting drug users and sexual risk behaviour among heterosexual men and women. The studies reported upon are largely from the developed world. As was noted in the discussion of the 'core groups' hypothesis in Chapter 2, there is a small but important literature of parallel anthropological studies from the Third World (more such work is urgently required) and such studies will also be referenced.

Sexual risk behaviour among men who have sex with men

Anal intercourse, for many gay men, does not have the central place in their sexual relationships that vaginal intercourse has in most heterosexual sexual relationships. In the UK Project Sigma study, a sample of 930 gay men recruited from non-agency settings such as bars, clubs and friendship networks, 15 per cent of those interviewed in 1987–88 had never engaged in anal intercourse (Davies et al., 1990); 20 per cent of those re-interviewed in 1991 had not engaged in anal intercourse between 1987 and 1991; moreover, only 33.1 per cent considered anal intercourse to be 'central, very, or quite important to their sexual repertoire' (Hickson et al., 1992a).

A common finding in a range of sociological studies of risk behaviour among men who have sex with men in the UK and elsewhere (Davies et al., 1993a; Kippax et al., 1993) is that risk behaviour is strongly associated with particular kinds of relationships with partners. Broadly speaking, penetrative sex occurs most frequently with a regular sexual partner and, as in heterosexual relationships, is seen as emblematic of intimacy, love and trust: sex with regular partners is much more likely to involve unsafe sex than sex with casual partners. Indeed, it may be something of a misnomer to designate anal sex as 'unsafe sex' when it occurs between two HIV-negative, mutually monogamous men; 43.7 per cent of those Project Sigma respondents interviewed in 1990 who were in relationships reported themselves to be monogamous (Hunt et al., 1992). In a longitudinal study of a large sample of US young gay and bisexual men, the best predictor of respondents changing over time from low- to high-risk behaviour was that of entering into a 'lover relationship' (Hays et al., 1992). A frequently observed pattern of gay relationships in the AIDS era is that of unsafe sex with a regular partner, with both partners also reporting safer sex with casual partners outside the relationship. For example:

> We screw each other but have safer sex with other people. This has been the case since we met. We both knew the realities of the risks. (quoted in Hickson et al., 1992b: 417)

Earlier, in Chapter 3, there was some discussion of the considerable falls in numbers of reported penetrative partners that occurred in the mid-1980s. For example, in the San Francisco Men's Health Study, the numbers of reports of receptive anal intercourse with two or more partners in the previous six months fell by 80 per cent between 1984 and 1987 (Winkelstein et al., 1988). This spectacular rate of change could not be maintained for a lengthy period and it was no surprise when studies conducted in the late 1980s reported that this downward trend was no longer apparent and that the trend had perhaps even undergone a slight reversal. Nevertheless, the fact that most unsafe sex occurs between regular homosexual partners has clearly played a large part in ensuring a fall in the numbers of new cases of HIV infection in the 'sexual intercourse between men' transmission category in many developed countries. In the UK, for example, the numbers of known new cases of HIV-1 transmitted by sexual intercourse between men fell from 1,430 cases in 1992 to 1,361 cases in 1993.

By no means all casual homosexual encounters are safer sexual encounters but, in any case, the restriction of unsafe sex to regular sexual partners would not in itself end epidemic spread. Every person who knows people living with AIDS and HIV has heard tragic histories of persons whose trust in their partner's fidelity was betrayed. But, more importantly, many gay men have more than one regular partner: 23.8 per cent of the Project Sigma respondents interviewed in 1990 who had regular partners reported more than one regular partner; 4 per cent reported five or more regular partners (Hickson et al., 1992b). Further, even those practising monogamy may only be practising serial monogamy: the median length of regular relationships reported in the 1990 Project Sigma interviews was 21 months (Hickson et al., 1992b). Some 'regular' partnerships are of very short duration (Fitzpatrick et al., 1989): although it may be the respondent's current intention to form a lasting relationship with their new partner, they may sometimes be guilty of romantic optimism.

Attempts to differentiate by socio-demographic variables those men practising safer sex and those practising unsafe sex have met with little success. Davies et al. (1992) have disputed the hypothesis that younger gay men are more likely than older men to practise unsafe sex. In a large sample of gay men attending the 1993 Lesbian and Gay Pride March in London, there was no association between either age or years of sexual experience and reports of protected or unprotected anal sex (Davies et al., 1993b). In contrast, one American study has shown an association between unprotected anal intercourse and the age of the respondent *after* controlling for the type of relationship reported (Jay et al., 1992), but this study was conducted on an unusual population, gay men entering a substance abuse programme. As was noted in the previous chapter, American data also show higher frequencies of anal intercourse among non-white gay men, but it is unclear how far this apparent ethnic difference may be an artefact of unexamined differences in behaviour based on wealth and status.

More surprising than the seeming absence of socio-demographic associations with unsafe same-gender sex is the lack of association with intoxication, especially given the popularity in Western cultures of accounts where intoxication diminishes the narrator's responsibility ('Don't blame me, I was pissed out of my skull'). Although Plant (1990) has reviewed a number of studies which do associate HIV-related risk behaviour with intoxication, a number of well-conducted studies of risk behaviour among men who have sex with men show no such association (for example, Weatherburn et al., 1992). This might be thought to be a consequence of the very strong association between unsafe sex and type of relationship (regular or casual), but two recent Australian studies of older and younger (15–21-year-old) gay men (Gold et al., 1991; Gold and Skinner, 1992) showed no association between unsafe sex and intoxication, even when unsafe casual sexual encounters were considered separately. Of course, this need not imply a similar absence of association between intoxication and heterosexual risk behaviour. While the lack of association between unsafe sex and intoxication may be surprising, the lack of association with knowledge about HIV transmission is readily comprehensible. All studies of men who have sex with men have shown very high levels of knowledge of HIV transmission, even among men under 21 years of age. As Fitzpatrick et al. (1989) have pointed out, this near-uniformity in high levels of HIV/AIDS knowledge has meant that tests of such knowledge have been poor discriminators of variations in risk behaviour.

A number of studies have attempted to explain risk behaviour by reference to beliefs about HIV/AIDS rather than to knowledge, attempting to trace variations in risk behaviour to variations in individuals' perceptions of the severity of the personal threat of HIV, to variations in the perceived efficacy of preventive action, and so on. This is the 'health beliefs' model and will be considered in more detail alongside other models of risk behaviour in Chapter 5. We can note here that the model has proved a poor predictor of risk behaviour in a large Chicago study of gay men (Joseph et al., 1987).

It is sometimes suggested that a perceptual element may help explain one supposed difference in risk behaviour among men who have sex with men, namely that between those who self-identify as gay and those who engage in same-gender sex but self-identify as bisexual or 'straight'. Thus the US Blood Donor Study Group identified and interviewed 209 HIV-positive male donors who reported sex with other men; those who self-identified as heterosexual or bisexual had lower perceptions of risk prior to donation than the gay-identified men – they did not see themselves as being in a 'risk group'. Moreover, those donors who both self-identified as heterosexual and also reported anal intercourse with a male partner in the previous year, were more likely than gay and bisexually identified respondents to have engaged in unprotected intercourse (Doll et al., 1992). Of course, the presumption of a causal relationship between perceptions of risk and risk behaviour may be unfounded: men who have sex with other men but self-identify as 'straight' would be less likely to perceive themselves as at risk, but they would also be less subject to the peer pressures within the gay constituency to practise safer sex. The relationships between sexual identity, identity disclosure, gay community involvement and unsafe sex are complex (see, for example, Kippax et al., 1993). In Kippax et al.'s Australian sample of men who had sex with men, 58 per cent of those who also reported sex with women said that all their female partners knew that they were 'bisexual'. Although Kippax et al. found that generally in their sample involvement with the gay community was important in promoting and sustaining safer sexual behaviour, that fraction of the sample who reported recent female partners had low gay community involvement, but they also reported adoption of protected sex with male partners to a degree equivalent to that reported by that fraction of the sample only reporting male partners. American data showing bisexual men engaging in higher levels of risk behaviour than gay-identified men has not always been confirmed by studies in other parts of the developed world (see the review by Boulton and Weatherburn, 1990).

As we have seen in Chapter 2, notions of homosexuality or bisexuality may be alien to some cultures in the Third World such as that of Brazil, where an active/passive distinction is more culturally salient. Indeed, the greater cultural diversity of American society may lie at the heart of US–UK differences in bisexual risk behaviour: certainly, among American men who have sex with men there are clear ethnic differences in sexual affiliations, with white men who have sex with men being more likely to self-identify as gay, Black men who have sex with men being more likely to self-identify as bisexual, and Hispanic men who have sex with men more likely to self-identify as heterosexual (Doll et al., 1992). Again it seems that local cultural differences in sexual practices and learned responses to the epidemic may be an important determinant of risk behaviour.

Male prostitution, while a less frequent phenomenon than female prostitution, may account for an important fraction of all unsafe same-gender sexual contacts. Male prostitution is a highly differentiated phenomenon: the call-man with his own flat and a 'book' of regular clients, packing for an extended trip to South America with a businessman client, is far removed from a crowd of jostling, half-drunk adolescents milling around the steps of a late-night public lavatory; among street-working male prostitutes, there are some men who have the same instrumental and businesslike orientation as their female street-prostitute colleagues, while others have a casual and haphazard approach that perhaps has more in common with juvenile delinquency than with female prostitution.

A number of local sociological studies in America, Britain and Europe have established that at least a substantial minority of male prostitutes (a majority in some local studies) are currently practising anal sex (protected or unprotected, as receptor or insertor or both) with at least some of their clients (Bloor et al., 1993a; Coutinho et al., 1988; Davies and Feldman, 1991; Elifson et al., 1993; Morse et al., 1991). As previously noted, the highest rates of anal sex are found in transvestite and transsexual prostitute populations (for example Elifson et al., 1990; Reckhart et al., 1993). Davies and Feldman detected a tendency for anal sex to be more common with 'regular' clients than with 'casual' clients, a finding that seemingly mirrors other data on how unsafe sex is associated with particular kinds of relationships.

However, the association of anal sex with regular clients may also be related to the greater likelihood that sex took place at the client's home: casual clients are less likely to take a prostitute to their homes and disrobing for anal sex is a hazardous venture in cars, parks and lavatory cubicles. In any case, anal sex was not confined to regular clients in Davies and Feldman's South Wales study, where 10 per cent of encounters with casual clients in the previous week had entailed anal sex (Davies and Feldman, 1991: 11).

Few male prostitutes undertake anal sex as a matter of volition; one might properly state that unsafe male commercial sex is indeed associated with particular kinds of relationships, but with particular kinds of *power* relationships (see the extended discussion in Chapter 5). Unsafe commercial sex is associated with client control (sometimes, indeed, with physical intimidation); safer commercial sex is associated with directive control of the encounter by the prostitute (Bloor et al., 1993a). Where male prostitutes are prepared, like female prostitutes, to state explicitly their terms and prices, then the interactional initiative is theirs; where they adopt a more passive stance, then whether or not unsafe sex takes place will be a matter for the client's discretion.

Most of the information available on clients of male prostitutes has been obtained indirectly from prostitutes, although there have been two valuable German interview studies, one with clients of German male prostitutes (Schrott-Ben Redjeb et al., 1992) and one with gay German sex tourists in Thailand (Wilke and Kleiber, 1992; see also Wirawan et al., 1992, on interviews with gay sex tourists in Bali). Just as male prostitution is a highly heterogeneous phenomenon, so also the clients of male prostitutes are a highly heterogeneous grouping. While some clients are clearly seeking a business relationship (fast, uncomplicated sex), others are contacting prostitutes as part of a partnership search, or as a partner substitute. It is commonly supposed that clients are 'closet' gay men or bisexual men without access to sexual partners through local gay subcultures. Certainly, such persons form one substantial component of the client population and it is possible that the comparative insulation of this group from peer gay pressure may help explain their relative lack of commitment to safer sex.

However, older gay-identified men with sexual preferences for younger partners also form a component of the client group; there is allegedly a paedophile component among gay sex tourists. The world of street prostitution, in particular, is one of ambiguity and potential violence. Perlongher (1987), a Brazilian ethnographer who has conducted a detailed study of the Brazilian 'miche' (male prostitute), suggests that some clients may find in the very risks of the encounter a potent erotic charge: for these clients, safety may equate with boredom. Unless such client preferences are contested by the prostitute, unsafe sex will result.

The location of the causes of unsafe commercial sex in the immediate situation of the sexual encounter has resonances with some research findings concerning unsafe private sexual encounters between men. Two Australian studies (Gold et al., 1991; Gold and Skinner, 1992) sought to compare reports from gay men of two contrasting recent occasions when they had engaged in safer (protected) and unsafe sex. While some of those factors which distinguished unsafe from safer sexual encounters have already been examined (type of relationship), and others were elements which respondents brought to the encounter (mood state, sexual desire), or which related to respondents' perceptions (inferences about the partner's likely HIV status), others again were what the authors termed 'situational factors', factors relating to the immediate situation of the sexual encounter. One such situational factor was a failure to communicate with their partner about whether or not they should practise safer sex; another factor was the use of, in the authors' phrase, 'dirty talk', which may have been interpreted by the partner as expressing a desire for unprotected intercourse. As in commercial sexual encounters, where the ambiguity of the situation is not dispelled by explicit discussion, the partner may be allowed to proceed by default to unsafe sex.

Other parallels between private and commercial same-gender sex relate to the possibility of intimidation into non-consensual unsafe sex, and to the influence of geographical location on sexual behaviour. With respect to the first of these possibilities, the Project Sigma study found that more than a quarter of 930 gay and bisexual respondents reported that they had been subjected to non-consensual sex at some point in their lives; 45 per cent of these had been forcibly anally penetrated (Hickson et al., 1994). Relatedly, male rape is a well-known hazard of male prostitution; Ritchie McMullen, an ex-prostitute and experienced care-worker, claimed that nearly all London's male prostitutes had suffered at least one rape (McMullen, 1990).

A second possibility concerns the sexual behaviour of gay men who 'cottage', that is, meet men for private sexual encounters at 'cottages', or public lavatories (in Glaswegian gay argot the practice is known as 'trawling' or 'bucking'; in America, cottages are known as 'tearooms'). Sexual behaviour in cottages is much influenced by the limited privacy afforded by the lavatories. Only a small proportion of sexual acts between cottagers involve anal penetration (Keogh et al., 1992) and most such anal intercourse occurs in that minority of instances where the cottagers retire to a partner's home (Davies et al., 1993a). Similarly, an ethnographic study of the sexual encounters that occurred in the cabins in Stockholm's popular gay porno video clubs (Hendriksson and Mansson, 1992) stressed that very few cases of anal sex were observed because of the limited privacy of the settings. The atypicality of penetrative sex among men who meet at 'cottages' or cruising grounds, such as public parks after dark, is partly compensated for by the relative frequency with which men resort to cottages, but only partly: in the Project Sigma data, respondents who sought casual partners in public places (i.e. pubs, clubs, cottages, cruising grounds, saunas, beaches, parties and the streets) went to cottages a mean number of 7.0 times per month but only averaged 1.6 penetrative partners a year through cottaging; in contrast, gay pubs were visited 5.2 times per month and resulted in 3.0 penetrative partners per year (Davies et al., 1993a: 157).

The public health achievements of the gay community (Coxon and Carballo, 1989 prefer the term 'constituency' to 'community', but accuracy must defer to convention) have been extraordinary. However, while anal penetration (like vaginal penetration) is associated with intimacy and trust, it is unlikely that anal penetration (protected or unprotected) will be eliminated from the sexual repertoires of men who have sex with men. This association of unsafe sex with a particular type of sexual relationship seems likely to continue to cause new cases of infection, at least in the medium term, with seropositive men infecting their seronegative regular partner(s). Yet the main epidemic threat lies not in unsafe sex with regular partners, but in unsafe sex with casual partners. As we have seen, the latter practices are reported only by a minority of men who have sex with men, but small numbers of men with large numbers of penetrative partners may have an epidemic impact out of all proportion to their numerical importance. Some of the research findings discussed above have suggested that unsafe sex in casual relationships may be associated with situational factors. This is a topic to which we shall return in discussing similar findings relating to other epidemiological transmission categories.

Syringe-sharing among injecting drug users

Just as there had been no UK survey of sexual behaviour prior to the HIV epidemic, so also there had been no UK social research on syringe-sharing, despite the fact that such sharing was known to be implicated in the spread of blood-borne infections such as hepatitis B. However, a pioneering American sociological study from 1970 (Howard and Borges, 1970) had long established that limited access to clean injecting equipment was not the sole reason for sharing among injectors. The establishment of syringe-exchange schemes has been an important component in the public health effort against HIV in every country where such exchanges have been permitted (Des Jarlais and Friedman, 1992) – they remain illegal in most states of the USA and in a number of other countries (for example Burma) with substantial epidemics of HIV among injecting drug users. Nevertheless, access to clean injecting equipment is a necessary, rather than a sufficient, condition for drug injectors to avoid needle-sharing. As Howard and Borges showed more than twenty years ago, needle-sharing does not occur randomly: it arises out of particular kinds of social relationships and carries particular social meanings for the injectors concerned, notably the signification of friendship with, and trust of, one's fellow injector(s). There is thus an arresting parallel with the above sociological research on men who have sex with men, indicating that risk behaviour is associated with particular kinds of social relationship and with feelings of intimacy and trust.

What was true in 1970 remains the case in the 1990s. Although there has been an enormous reduction in syringe-sharing since the early years of the HIV epidemic (a reduction that parallels the reduction in risk behaviour in the gay community), the syringe-sharing that still occurs remains socially patterned, associated for the most part with close friendships, sexual relationships and family ties. Table 4.1 illustrates this point. Derived from interview data collected in 1991 from 535 Glasgow injectors, the table shows respondents' reports of their relationships with all persons from whom they borrowed injecting equipment in the previous six months. Those respondents who had borrowed others' used equipment were much more likely to have borrowed from their immediate social circle (regular sexual partner, close friend or family member) than from a comparative stranger: 75 per cent of all recent sharing partners were from the injectors' immediate social circles (Bloor et al., 1994).

Similar, but less marked, evidence of social discrimination among sharing partners is to be found in the same group of respondents'

Table 4.1   *Persons from whom respondents had ever borrowed injecting equipment in the previous six months*

Immediate social circle	
1. Close friend	98
2. Regular sexual partner	53
3. Family member	23
Others	
4. Dealer	12
5. Fellow prisoner	12
6. Someone they did not know	12
7. Someone in the street	11
8. Shooting gallery	10
Total reports	231

No. of respondents: 535

reports of lending of their equipment to others. It should be appreciated that the term 'sharing' conflates a number of different activities that carry with them varying risks of infection: lending of equipment carries less risk for the lender than borrowing, since not all equipment will be returned and not all returned equipment will be re-used without sterilisation; and sharing a 'hit' dissolved in blood drawn up into the syringe clearly carries more risk than the re-use of previously discarded and rinsed (but not sterilised) injecting equipment. It is not surprising that some studies (including the Glasgow study above) have found injectors more willing to lend than to borrow: mutual obligations of friendship may make it difficult for injectors to refuse friends desperate for a hit:

> my pals ask me sometimes if they havenae got any works [equipment]. I give them then. I couldnae knock them back because I know they'd not refuse me. (quoted in McKeganey and Barnard, 1992: 42)

McKeganey and Barnard's ethnography lists six possible influences on sharing (1992: 36–45). Three such influences have already been mentioned: access to clean equipment; the nature of the relationship between the sharing individuals; and local cultural norms which stress obligations to help out neighbours and friends, norms which frequently have great force in those UK working-class neighbourhoods where the 1980s explosion in injecting drug use appears to have been concentrated (Parker et al., 1988). The other three influences are: a seemingly compelling need to inject, an assessment of limited risk, and inadvertent sharing.

Injected drugs vary in their physiological addictiveness: for example the most commonly injected drugs in some places (Sweden, South Wales) are amphetamines, not opiates, and are not thought to be physiologically addictive at all. A few opiate injectors report a determination to postpone their hit until they can find clean injecting equipment, and a few will opt to snort, swallow or smoke their drugs instead, despite the lesser effectiveness of such methods compared to injection. But many opiate injectors freely report their willingness to use others' equipment if they are desperate for a hit.

Some injectors report a readiness to share selectively with those fellow injectors whom they judge to be unlikely to be infected. This judgement may be based merely on the appearance of health, but is also frequently based on long acquaintance. Sharing may be based on calculation, but it may also be based on trust. The assessment that one's sharing partner is a limited risk thus has close affinities with the earlier statement that risk behaviour is influenced by particular kinds of social relationships. Between two sexual partners who are injectors, for example, the male partner may be willing to share equipment because he calculates that his partner is unlikely to infect him because she is sharing with no one else, while the female partner may be willing to share as a demonstration and consequence of intimacy and trust. And who is to say that the calculation that one's partner is unlikely to be infected is not trust by another name?

Inadvertent sharing probably occurs most frequently when injectors mix up each other's equipment. Such mix-ups are readily envisaged where injectors hit up together but each has his or her own equipment; the likelihood of accidents may be increased where injectors are using barbiturates and other drugs which may impair their clarity of thought or memory. It should also be recalled that injectors, like medical and nursing personnel, are subject to needle-stick injury.

The issue of access to sterile equipment has been dealt with so far only in terms of syringe-exchanges and requires a broader treatment. Lack of access may, of course, occur even in areas where exchanges and sales points abound – they may be shut at the time the injector wishes to hit up. (The automated syringe dispensers pioneered in some European cities are unlikely to catch on in the vandalism-and-vigilante cultures of British and American cities.) But the injector's access to equipment may be deliberately restricted. Not all drug injectors in prison continue to inject, but those who do are much more likely to share equipment than drug injectors 'at large': interviews with English ex-prisoners indicated that only 22 per cent of injecting drug users injected while in prison, but three-quarters of these had shared equipment (Turnbull et al., 1990). As McKeganey and Barnard (1992: 45) have indicated, even those prisoners who have no wish to share may be intimidated into loaning and then re-using their equipment: the social relationships that pattern sharing embrace fear and domination as well as intimacy and trust.

Syringe-sharing among prisoners is of particular epidemiological importance because prisons mix together drug users who, outside prison, normally only share equipment with their immediate social circles. These social circles are then infected in turn by ex-prisoners on their release: drug-injector prisoners may approximate to an epidemiological 'core group', as discussed in Chapter 2. Hence the public health effort to control HIV outbreaks in prisons, such as that mounted at the Glenochil Young Offenders Institution in Scotland in 1993.

While the problem of syringe-sharing in prisons is well understood, there is less recognition that the same phenomenon may be found in residential drug treatment institutions (Bloor et al., 1989). Not all residents of such institutions are strongly motivated to achieve abstinence: it is commonplace, for example, for a solicitor to advise a drug injector client to enrol on a drug treatment programme prior to an upcoming court case. Under such circumstances institutions dedicated to abstinence may become the innocent and unwitting agents of epidemic spread.

The various influences on sharing behaviour outlined above have a disproportionate impact on different sub-groups of the drug-injecting population. The association of syringe-sharing with intimacy and trust may account for the high levels of syringe-sharing among female injectors. In the previously mentioned Glasgow interview study, behavioural and socio-demographic correlates of sharing were mathematically modelled (Frischer et al., 1993): the three strongest correlates of syringe-sharing were the frequency with which the respondent injected, gender, and lack of a fixed address. Since there are far fewer female injectors than male injectors (the estimated gender ratio among Glasgow injectors was 2.6 males to one female – Frischer et al., 1992a), the chances of a female injector having a fellow injector as a regular sexual partner are much greater than for a male injector, there being fewer female injectors around. Consequently, there is more scope for female injectors to share injecting equipment with their sexual partners: more of *their* partners will be fellow injectors (Barnard, 1992).

The association between lack of a fixed address and increased levels of sharing may be explicable by the possibility that both factors are indicative of a chaotic lifestyle. However, an alternative explanation may lie in the fact that those injectors with no fixed address and dependent on others for accommodation may find it difficult to resist pressure to share from other residents in the same accommodation. Donoghoe et al. (1991) report that syringe-sharers in their sample were more likely than non-sharers to live in shared accommodation.

The association between reported sharing and reported frequency of injecting is an important but sometimes overlooked feature of drug injectors' risk behaviour. Clearly, other things being equal, an injector who injects very frequently is more likely to report some sharing than an injector who injects on an occasional basis. However, this 'frequency' effect is sometimes partly obscured by the cross-cutting influence of the type of drug injected on propensity to share. For example, as stated previously, the most commonly injected drugs in South Wales are probably amphetamines rather than opiates. Amphetamines are commonly used on social occasions in the local youth culture and so their injection may often be associated with syringe-sharing. However, amphetamines are not physiologically addictive and thus are unlikely to be injected on a daily basis; in a sample of Welsh drug injectors attending a syringe-exchange scheme only 36 per cent injected more frequently than five times per week (Stimson et al., 1992). Opiate users may have a lesser propensity to share than amphetamine users on each occasion that they inject, but the fact that opiate injectors inject far more frequently means that they will report more syringe-sharing per week or per month. In contrast to Stimson et al.'s Welsh sample, more than 90 per cent of the Glasgow sample above (who were largely opiate injectors) injected at least once per day. Not surprisingly, they also reported higher rates of syringe-sharing over time.

Barbiturate injectors may inject less frequently than opiate injectors but their propensity to share may possibly be greater because of the perceptual changes associated with barbiturate use (Klee et al., 1990a): no one who has watched Temazepam injectors barrelling off walls and falling down in the road can be very sanguine about their ability to practise HIV-risk reduction. However, this barbiturates–opiates distinction is of less value than the amphetamines–opiates distinction, since many barbiturates injectors are in fact poly-drug users: for instance, Temazepam ('Jellies' or 'Eggs') and other barbiturates may be injected occasionally by regular opiate injectors who may be unable to score any opiates and seek to dull with barbiturates the pain and anxiety of temporary opiate withdrawal.

Inadvertent risk behaviour by Temazepam users notwithstanding, it is clear that there has been a sharp reduction in syringe-sharing among drug injectors in the late 1980s and 1990s. The UK government's revised 'Day Report' rather stiffly stated that 'the occurrence of such a change in a group normally resistant to health education' was 'surprising' (PHLS Working Group, 1993: S15) but it was clearly borne out by epidemiological evidence of a fall in new HIV infections among UK drug injectors; the Working Group went on to downwardly revise its previous projections of future AIDS cases among injectors.

Table 4.2 illustrates this reduction in risk behaviour in the Glasgow study. The reductions in both borrowing and lending were statistically significant ($z^2 = 19.1$, p = <0.01; $z^2 = 6.9$, p = <0.05). At the same time the average number of persons from whom syringes were received fell from 3.7 to 2.7 and the average number of persons to whom syringes were passed on fell from 7.6 to 5.8 persons (t = 2.1, p = <0.05) (Bloor et al., 1994). What is more, it seems likely that these reductions in risk behaviour had already begun prior to 1990: in 1988 for example, 76 per cent of the Scottish respondents in a UK study of injectors reported that they had shared in the previous *four weeks* (Stimson et al., 1988a).

This fall in risk behaviour, similarly documented in other studies of injecting drug users around the world, is a major public health achievement on a par with that achieved by the gay community. However, readers may be somewhat puzzled about how a *reduction* in risk behaviour (dramatic or not) can be effective in securing the seeming stabilisation of HIV prevalence noted in the previous chapter: the logically minded might reasonably object that, if HIV has already entered a local population, then a mere reduction in risk behaviour (as opposed to complete cessation of risk behaviour) would slow, but not halt, HIV spread. This conundrum will be examined in more detail.

Table 4.2 *Changes in reported syringe-sharing, 1990–91*

	1990	1991
Percentage of respondents who report never injecting with used equipment given by someone else ('borrowed') in the previous six months	287 (57%)	377 (70%)
Percentage of respondents who report never giving/ selling/lending used equipment in the previous six months	213 (42%)	288 (54%)
Total no. of respondents	503	535

Source: Bloor et al., 1994

One possible explanation for the stabilisation of HIV prevalence lies in what has previously been referred to as 'epidemiological saturation' (Blower, 1991): it is suggested that local levels of infection have stabilised because all those seriously at risk have already become infected. This is an argument stressing behavioural heterogeneity rather than behavioural change, with local stabilisation occurring at the saturation point when all of the high risk sub-group of local drug injectors are infected. A difficulty with this view is the fact that HIV-prevalence stabilisation seems to have occurred at very different levels between different cities. Among New York drug injectors prevalence has stabilised at 47 per cent (Des Jarlais et al., 1991) and among Edinburgh drug injectors prevalence has stabilised at around 20 per cent (Bath et al., 1993); in contrast, HIV prevalence among San Francisco drug injectors has stabilised at below 10 per cent (Sorensen et al., 1989) and among Glasgow injectors it is less than 2 per cent (Taylor et al., 1994). It is difficult to see why saturation should occur at such different levels of prevalence in different cities.

Another possible reason for stabilisation was touched upon in the previous chapter, namely attrition in the numerator population: that is, the disappearance from local populations of drug injectors of those who are HIV positive. HIV-positive drug injectors have higher mortality rates than uninfected injectors (Frischer et al., 1992b; Galli et al., 1991) – seemingly largely through overdoses rather than through HIV-related illnesses. And it may be that they are also more likely than other injectors to cease injecting (Frischer et al., 1992c), particularly if they are offered oral methadone by service-providers. Consequently, a steady trickle of new infections among drug injectors is perfectly compatible with stable HIV prevalence: those newly infected merely serve to replace the artefactual attrition from the earlier infected population (Bloor et al., 1994).

Biological explanations have also been advanced for these inter-city differences in prevalence levels. It has been thought that an explanation may lie in local differences in genetic susceptibility to infection, but this too seems implausible; although there is evidence to show that there are indeed genetic differences in susceptibility (for example Louie et al., 1991), no substantial differences in the gene pool between adjacent cities such as Edinburgh and Glasgow can be expected. Another possibility that has been canvassed is that differing viral strains of different virulence may be predominant in different cities. This too seems unlikely to be the case when cities are as close together as Edinburgh and Glasgow and it is known that drug injectors from both cities mingle together at dealing points, in prisons and in drug treatment centres. In any case, recent work in the field of molecular epidemiology seems to indicate that all the main strains of the virus are all widely distributed across the globe.

It thus seems clear that the stabilisation of HIV prevalence among drug injectors relates to risk reduction rather than epidemiological saturation, genetic susceptibility or viral strain. Stabilisation has occurred at different levels of prevalence in different cities because the epidemic began in some cities earlier than others and had therefore spread further in some cities before risk reduction occurred. Stabilisation occurred despite the fact that risk behaviour was reduced rather than eliminated. This happened for two reasons: firstly, HIV is only inefficiently transmitted (recall the data from Chapter 3 concerning the very low infection ratio in cases of exposure through occupational needlestick injuries) – HIV is transmitted much less readily by syringe-sharing than, say, hepatitis B; and secondly, syringe-sharing is socially patterned, with little opportunity for the virus to cross over from one limited social network of injectors to another. Under these circumstances, the resultant trickle of new cases of infection may be cancelled out by differential attrition in the numerator population (higher mortality rates and cessation rates among the HIV-positive injectors) resulting in stable prevalence rates in cross-sectional studies (as opposed to follow-up studies) of injectors.

This stabilisation of HIV prevalence is not confined to cities of the developed world. It has also been demonstrated among drug injectors in cities in the developing world like Bangkok. However, the parallel changes in risk behaviour among injectors in Bangkok have only been achievable through the provision of increased access to sterile injecting equipment. Every developing country on a drug trafficking route, from Nigeria to Nagaland, eventually finds itself with an indigenous population of drug injectors. In some of these countries access to sterile injecting equipment remains restrictive; in Myanmar (Burma) for example, the sale of syringes is illegal and the tribesmen in the hills are reported to pay for the use of a common syringe from a fellow-villager – a procedure which amounts to serial anonymous sharing and which has been associated with a very rapid increase in HIV prevalence to astonishing levels in some localities of 80 to 95 per cent (Stimson, 1994b). Further sudden increases in prevalence must be expected in other developing countries where drug trafficking occurs but access to syringes is limited.

Even in the developed world the current (partly artefactual) stability of HIV prevalence among drug injectors may be a transitory achievement. This fear has its roots, not in a possible future reversion to increased sharing among current injectors (although any increase in the present prison population should be viewed with some alarm), but rather in future possible changes in the injector population. Past changes have not been readily predicted and have thrown up new populations of injectors who have had to learn anew the lessons of harm reduction painfully learned by earlier groups of injectors. In South Wales, for example, a limited epidemic of heroin injecting in the early 1980s in Cardiff and Newport was succeeded in the late 1980s by a wave of amphetamine injection among a quite different younger group of injectors in the Valleys. Most recently, there have been reports of steroid injection among a third local sub-population, this time bodybuilders (Pates and Temple, 1992; Korkia and Stimson, 1993). Reports of increased levels of syringe-sharing may thus occur, not through risk-reversion among the existing injector population, but through population replacement.

Where HIV infection newly enters an injector population among whom syringe-sharing is extensive, then there are reasons to suppose that epidemic spread will be rapid. It is thought that the transmissibility of the virus is greatest when the infected person is him/herself first infected, before they have developed antibodies to the virus. Once antibodies are developed, transmissibility is greatly reduced and only increases slowly again as the infected person develops AIDS and their viral load thus increases. As a consequence, the characteristic pattern of HIV infection among injecting drug users may be one of sudden explosions of infection, with the virus spreading rapidly through linked sharing networks of injectors before antibodies develop and transmissibility declines. After antibodies develop, the low levels of transmissibility may be insufficient to sustain further substantial epidemic spread where substantial risk reduction has taken place, but some risk behaviour still occurs. Sudden epidemic explosions like those of Edinburgh and Bangkok may thus be a characteristic pattern and further explosions of infection are always a potential hazard where syringe-sharing continues to occur. On a small scale, the sudden rise in infections among injectors at Glenochil Young Offenders Institution in Scotland in the summer of 1993 is testimony to the continuing fragility of current public health achievements in the fight against the epidemic among injecting drug users.

Sexual risk behaviour among heterosexual men and women

Of the 8 to 10 million adults world-wide estimated by the World Health Organisation in 1991 to be infected with HIV, three-quarters had contracted the virus by heterosexual transmission. This is a proportion likely to rise, not just because heterosexual transmission is likely to be of increasing relative importance in the developed world, but also because most new cases of HIV infection will be in developing countries, where heterosexual transmission has always been the predominant pattern. The route whereby the virus first becomes locally established may vary: in South America, male prostitution appears to be playing an important early role since many clients also have female partners; in South-East Asia, injecting drug use may have been of initial importance (this is a matter of current dispute). Once the virus has been established in a developing country, heterosexual transmission rapidly becomes the main viral transmission route. The looming prospect of a major epidemic in the Indian sub-continent would further emphasise the relative importance of heterosexual transmission.

The reasons are not fully understood why heterosexual transmission has played such a differentially important part (to date) in HIV transmission in the developing world compared to the developed world. Part of the answer certainly lies in the higher rates of other sexually transmitted diseases, which (as was seen earlier) may both increase susceptibility to infection and also increase the HIV-positive person's infectiousness through genital ulceration. Part of the answer almost certainly does *not* lie in a high prevalence of heterosexual anal intercourse. Although heterosexual anal intercourse is reportedly commonplace in South America, it is seemingly unknown (and regarded as either risible or shocking) in many parts of Africa. Homosexual 'mine marriages' were reportedly once common among South African mine workers, who were forbidden to leave the mine compounds to visit women in the townships, but the sexual activity that occurred was normally 'metsha', insertion of the penis between the thighs, rather than anal penetration (Moodie, 1988). The use of herbs to dry the vagina (thus supposedly increasing male sexual pleasure but also increasing genital ulceration) has been suggested as an alternative candidate practice to heterosexual anal intercourse in amplifying viral transmissibility

(Nyirenda-Meya, 1992), but this practice seems to be of local rather than continental significance.

What remains unclear is whether rates of partner change and patterns of partner change between the developing and developed world may also be important components in an explanation for the different character of the epidemic. Systematic data on partner change in the developing world are unavailable. Instead of such systematic data, we have access to a range of anthropological accounts of local sexual behaviour, although there are clearly numerous problems in treating these heterogeneous local studies as if they were directly comparable.

One of the few authors to have attempted an overview of these anthropological accounts is Larson (1989). She points out that sexual mixing patterns differ sharply between patrilineal societies (where property is inherited through the male line of descent and where a wife joins a husband's kin at marriage) and matrilineal societies (where property passes to the son from the maternal uncle and where a wife remains part of her own family after marriage). In matrilineal societies, divorce is easier for women: they can look to their family of origin for economic support and they frequently also have the right to own land or retain the fruits of their agricultural labour – such women find it easier to quit an unsatisfactory marriage. Such economic independence for women tends to be accompanied by a degree of equality between the sexes in sexual mixing, with both men and women taking several lovers simultaneously or serially. In patrilineal societies, the dissolution of marriage occurs less frequently since divorced women lack alternative means of economic support and since the husband's kin will be loath to return the woman's bride-price. In such societies, pre-marital and extra-marital sexual relations involve small numbers of prostitutes and a large and overlapping male clientele. It is in societies of the latter type that HIV seems to spread most quickly.

However, Larson has also shown that, while cultural differences may be of some utility in explaining differing HIV prevalences, economic factors may often be more salient. She points out that the differences in HIV prevalence between Kigali in Rwanda (higher prevalence) and Kinshasa in Zaire (lower prevalence) may be traceable to the lack of economic opportunities for women in Kigali other than prostitution. Rwandan mores allow married women as well as men to have extra-marital relations with partners in specific kinship categories, but the absence of economic opportunities for women in the capital, Kigali, produced (prior to the civil war) a considerable imbalance of the sexes with 157 men to every 100 women in the 20 to 39 age-group in urban Rwanda. In Zaire, in contrast, the limping but diversified economy offers many more opportunities for women, particularly in market trading; as a result there is no urban sexual imbalance in population, with

98 men to every 100 women aged 20–44 years. Prostitution is by no means absent in Kinshasa, but the higher proportion of economically independent women may account for the much greater proportion of extra-marital contacts outside prostitution in Kinshasa than in Kigali. Larson cites epidemiological studies to show that 78 per cent of a sample of married men with AIDS in Kigali reported at least one contact with a prostitute, while only a third of a comparable group of Kinshasa male AIDS sufferers reported a prostitute contact. The latter group did, however, report an average of four extra-marital partners per year. Prostitution is associated with limited economic opportunities for African women (Robertson, 1984) and with urban gender imbalances.

In sum, very high rates of migration to the cities (Larson cites UN data showing annual increases in East African city populations of 7 per cent in the 1970s and 1980s) have combined with cultural mores of patrilineal societies to create patterns of sexual mixing that facilitate the very rapid transmission of STDs, namely the widespread recourse to prostitutes by male migrants with absent rural wives. This returns us to the 'core groups' hypothesis discussed in Chapter 2. As was noted previously, this hypothesis may be termed anthropologically naive since it fails to take into account the cultural diversity of Africa. The 'core groups' hypothesis may fit very well the patterns of sexual mixing found in some cities, but in other African cities private extra-marital sexual encounters may be more widespread and so commercial extra-marital encounters may be proportionately less important.

There has also been a number of anthropological studies of prostitution in African societies. Day (1988) has provided an overview of these studies, which both emphasises the rich diversity of prostitution practice and serves incidentally to qualify further the 'core groups' hypothesis. As we have already seen, it is by no means universal for all prostitutes to have large numbers of different clients: in some parts of Africa prostitutes may provide food and lodgings for clients with whom they may form long-standing but non-exclusive liasons. And studies of prostitution in the Gambia and the Lake Kariba area of Zimbabwe have shown their research subjects to be very locally mobile (indeed the majority of Gambian prostitutes were from neighbouring Senegal and Guinea-Bissau), suggesting that long-distance lorry-driver clients may be locally superfluous in linking local prostitute populations in a chain of HIV infection (Pickering et al., 1992).

When a Ugandan clinic nurse remonstrated with a male patient who was re-attending with a new sexually transmitted disease he replied: 'The bull is known by his scars.' However, there is some evidence that attitudes which link STDs with sexual prowess are changing and clients are showing greater readiness to wear condoms in commercial sexual encounters. A large number of local peer education programmes have been set up to mobilise changes in prostitution practice. One such pro-gramme in the Cameroons distributed over a million condoms in two years (Ikonga et al., 1992).

Nevertheless, there are a number of reasons why unsafe commercial sex is still practised. There remain some areas, particularly rural areas, where condoms are not readily available: in the Gambian study prosti-tutes reported using condoms with 80 per cent of their clients in urban areas, but when they worked the markets at outlying villages the per-centage dropped to 53 per cent (Pickering et al., 1992). Moreover, the HIV/AIDS campaigns adopted by a number of African governments have chosen to emphasise chastity outside marriage (the so-called 'zero grazing' approach) rather than the practice of safer sex; the former health education approach, in the European experience at least, has proved less effective than safer sex campaigns (Wellings, 1992). And relatedly, even the most vigorous peer-education campaign among prostitutes may be ineffective when prostitutes are economically depen-dent on uncooperative clients: the prostitute–client power relationship is at its most unequal where the prostitute is dependent on gifts or money from a few long-standing clients; as was seen in Chapter 2, sex tourists from the developed world are also infrequent condom users. Finally, prostitutes in the developing world, like their sisters elsewhere, rarely use condoms with their boyfriends. The boyfriends of the Gambian prostitutes studied by Pickering and her colleagues (1992) frequently had jobs in the bars where the women worked and 'rou-tinely' complained of symptoms of STDs. As Day et al. (1988) have suggested in the UK context, prostitute women may in fact be most at risk of HIV infection from their boyfriends. And since many of these relationships are transitory and non-exclusive, the barmen/boyfriends may act as agents of cross-infection – an old story: 'If a man be burnt with a harlot, and do meddle with another woman . . . he shall burn the woman that he shall meddle withal' (Boord, 1547).

In the developed world the heterosexual epidemic has been much more slow-building, due to a number of factors. Firstly, there is the absence, in the UK, of certain factors which have amplified the epi-demic in Africa and elsewhere, namely the lack of an epidemic role for female prostitution and the low prevalence of other STDs which increase infectiousness and (possibly also) susceptibility to HIV infec-tion. Secondly, local rates of sexual partner change and local patterns of sexual mixing may be such that transmission rates will be low.

Taking first the issue of prostitution practice, it is one of the ironies of the HIV epidemic that the public health has been preserved by the efforts of one of the most vilified and marginalised groups in society. Prostitutes in the UK and many other countries have long sought to practise safer commercial sex, not just to protect themselves from

STDs, but also to provide a symbolic barrier between themselves and their clients. While the condom barrier is there, women may feel that they have not been fully penetrated and that a clear difference exists between their private and their commercial sexual contacts (one reason why it is difficult for prostitute women to protect themselves from infection by their boyfriends, who may themselves be drug injectors – Day et al., 1988; McKeganey and Barnard, 1992).

The well-known association between female injecting drug use and female prostitution led to fears early on in the HIV epidemic that HIV-positive drug-injecting prostitutes would spread infection among their clients; it was supposed that the need to feed an addictive habit would lead drug injectors to succumb to clients who refused protected sex and/or who offered higher prices for unprotected sex. Hard evidence for this supposition has always been difficult to find. It is true that samples of clients report more unprotected commercial sex than samples of prostitutes: 17 per cent of a Glasgow sample (Barnard et al., 1993) and 9 per cent of a Manchester sample (Faugier et al., 1993) reported unprotected vaginal sex at their *last* prostitute encounter, whereas studies of UK prostitute samples have reported that 75 per cent or more of women report that *all* vaginal sex with clients is protected (for example Day, 1988). However, any tendency for drug-injecting prostitutes to undertake more unprotected commercial sex than non-injectors is probably related to their tendency to work longer hours to boost their earnings. In a Glasgow study of street prostitution where 70 per cent of the women were drug injectors, those women worked the streets on more nights and for longer hours than non-injectors (Bloor et al., 1991c). Factors other than drug use are likely to prove more salient in determining whether commercial sex is protected or not, for example whether or not the client was a regular customer, the type of prostitution engaged in (street-work, hostess-work, escort agency, massage parlour, brothel), and client intimidation. The most that can be said for a supposed association between drug use and unsafe commercial sex is that the use of certain drugs (most notably barbiturates like Temazepam) may so incapacitate prostitutes that they are quite incapable of insisting on condom use; but note that alcoholic intoxication is a related hazard for non-injecting prostitutes.

A related fear, that of the 'drug-crazed' female addict ready to take any risk for her next fix, has surfaced in respect of crack-addicted prostitutes in the United States, where the properties of the drug itself (short high, intense withdrawal suffering) are said to drive women to run great risks of HIV infection, despite the fact that the drug is usually smoked not injected. This has been thought to be the explanation for higher HIV prevalence rates among crack-addicted prostitutes in some studies (for example Golden et al., 1990). However, this too may be a false supposition, since many US crack addicts will ward off crack withdrawal symptoms by injecting opiates, with the associated likelihood that their higher HIV prevalence rates are the result of syringe-sharing rather than unsafe commercial sex. And, once again, women prostituting to support a crack addiction may be relatively more vulnerable to HIV infection simply because they are working longer hours and having sex with more clients.

It is believed that drug injectors working as prostitutes are at risk of HIV infection through their syringe-sharing rather than their commercial sexual behaviour. An EU cross-national study of prostitution found that the highest rates of HIV infection among prostitutes were in those countries of Southern Europe where the rates of HIV infection were highest among injecting drug users. A London study, which compared HIV prevalence rates between prostitute female injectors and non-prostitute female injectors, found no differences in rates (Rhodes et al., 1993).

The ability of prostitutes to practise safer sex with clients is associated with the women's directive control of the encounter (Barnard, 1993; McKeganey et al., 1990). In contrast to many of the male prostitutes practising unsafe commercial sex, prostitute women maintained interactional control of the encounter by demanding prior payment and by explicit statements of what acts they would perform at what prices. The use of the term 'business' in the street-cry that proclaims their prostitution ('Looking for business?') is an unintentional reflection of the women's brisk and purposive interactional manner:

> I was standing talking with a prostitute when a man slowly walked past. Seeing this, the woman turned round and asked him if he was looking for business. He didn't appear to speak much English, but he clearly was and asked about prices. 'Aye, well it's £10 in a motor and £25 in a flat.' He said he had no car, to which she replied, 'It'll have to be in a lane then.' He then asked, 'With or without Durex?' She didn't understand him at first, then she said, 'Oh no, it'll have to be with Durex unless you wank yourself off and I'll let you have a feel of me for £15.' (Barnard, 1993: 690)

Prostitutes in the developed world have established strategic relations with clients that enable them to practise safer commercial sex. But prostitutes in the developing world have difficulty establishing similar relations with developed world clients: the economic divide between the parties is perhaps too great. The phenomenon of 'sex tourism' may well be of more importance in stoking a heterosexual epidemic in the developed world than the phenomenon of local (developed world) prostitution. Before 1989 there were only two reports in England and Wales of known HIV infection following heterosexual exposure in Thailand; in 1991 and 1992 there were a total of seventeen such reports (Noone et al., 1992). Low levels of condom use were reported in interviews with German sex tourists in Bangkok (see Chapter 2). Client resistance to condom use was associated with client reluctance to view their relationships as commercial in character: many clients would consort with a single prostitute for the duration of their holiday and preferred to view the relationship as a 'holiday romance' (Wilke and Kleiber, 1991).

The volume of sex tourism is difficult to gauge. Few national sexual surveys have asked respondents questions about commercial sexual contacts abroad; the Swiss national telephone survey data were cited in Chapter 3. Wilke and Kleiber estimated that there were 40,000 to 50,000 German sex tourists per year visiting Bangkok, which itself is only one of a string of developing world sex tourism destinations – others are Bali, Brazil, the Dominican Republic, the Gambia, Hong Kong, the Philippines, and Sri Lanka.

Information on the size of the client population for developed world prostitution has been very limited until recently. The UK's NATSSAL study reports only 1.8 per cent of male respondents paying for sex with a woman in the previous five years (Johnson et al., 1994). Relatedly, socio-demographic data on clients are difficult to obtain: it will be no surprise that those who seek anonymous sex are sometimes reluctant respondents and the different sub-categories of prostitution work (street prostitution, call girls, massage parlours, escort agencies, club hostess work, brothels, etc.) may attract a differentiated clientele. Studies have thus sought to minimise bias by recruiting client respondents from a range of different sources – genito-urinary medicine clinics, direct recruitment of clients at prostitution sites and telephone interviews with respondents recruited by press advertisements. UK studies indicate that the majority of clients are married men living with their partners; safer sex is rarely reported with the clients' private sexual partners (Barnard et al., 1992). Men in white-collar employments appear to be over-represented among UK clients (Faugier et al., 1993). It might be thought that men whose employments require overnight absences are provided with more opportunities for commercial sexual contacts. However, the NATSSAL study did not find that job-related overnight absence was related to increased numbers of sexual partners among male respondents (Johnson et al., 1994). In some countries, notably Japan (Vorakitphokatorn and Cash, 1992), the offer of commercial sexual services is sometimes a component of 'corporate entertainment' of executives.

It has already been suggested that the 'core groups' hypothesis may be of locally variable importance in understanding the developing world epidemic, with other factors such as urban demography, development economics and cultural influences on sexual mixing patterns all playing important roles. It can now be seen that 'core groups' have played only a small part in the heterosexual HIV epidemic in the developed world and that has been partly through the phenomenon of sex tourism. Rather, the widespread practice by developed world prostitutes of safer commercial sex has served to restrict the spread of both HIV and of other STDs which amplify the infectiousness and susceptibility of partners to HIV infection. However, aside from commercial sexual encounters, rates of private unprotected sexual contact and partner change may also influence the course of the heterosexual epidemic and it is to studies of such partner change that we shall now turn.

At the start of the epidemic, policymakers were surprised and disconcerted to discover that the only data available on rates of sexual contact were the 'Kinsey Reports', based on American volunteer samples from the 1940s (Kinsey et al., 1948, 1953). Large-scale funding for pure or 'blue skies' social science research on sexual behaviour had never previously been available and now that information was urgently required for policy purposes the research work would have to be begun from scratch. In many countries plans were hurriedly laid for surveys to remedy this lacuna. The first survey to be completed was in Norway in 1988 (Sundet et al., 1988); British work was delayed by funding difficulties and the main survey of the NATSSAL study could not be begun until 1990. The first results of the study were published in the journal, *Nature*, at the end of 1992 (Johnson et al., 1992) and appeared in book form in 1994 (Johnson et al., 1994; Wellings et al., 1994).

The NATSSAL survey may justifiably be described as a model of good survey research practice in study design, sampling practice, survey instrument design and interviewer training. But, as the authors themselves note, suspicion about bias is readily voiced when the research subject is as sensitive as sexual behaviour. The sample surveyed was a household sample, with a consequent tendency for injecting drug users to be under-sampled as they are more likely than their peers to be in prison, in residential drug treatment or homeless. But aside from this limited sampling difficulty, it appears that any bias present is likely to be non-response bias rather than reporting bias or sampling bias: that is, that any bias stems from the differential likelihood of some sub-groups of the population refusing to respond, rather from the differential likelihood of some sub-groups mis-reporting their behaviour. The achieved response rate of 63.3 per cent was comparable with other surveys of sexual behaviour (like the Norwegian survey); men in the older age-groups were under-represented, but this appears to be less a consequence of direct refusal than a difficulty interviewers had in contacting some segments of the sample (Johnson et al., 1994).

Particular interest attaches to the NATSSAL findings on rates of heterosexual partner change and condom use. The mean rates of partner change were rather low: the mean number of heterosexual partners in the previous year was 1.2 for the men and 1.0 for the women (Johnson et al., 1992). Even in the youngest age-group the means were only 1.4 for the men and 1.0 for the women (see Johnson et al., 1990, for possible reasons for the lack of symmetry in gender responses). In a multiple regression analysis designed to identify those sub-groups of the population more likely to report multiple partners, the dominant influences on multiple partnerships for both men and women were those of age and marital status: the young and those previously married or single (including those cohabiting) were those most likely to report multiple partners in the previous year. There was also a small social class effect, with respondents in the two highest of the five occupational classes being more likely to report multiple partners. And finally, those reporting first intercourse before the age of 16 were also more likely to report more recent multiple partners (Johnson et al., 1994). In respect of condom use, only 25.9 per cent of women in the NATSSAL sample had used condoms in the past year; even in the youngest age-group (16–24-year-olds), only 41.8 per cent had used a condom in the past year. The implication of the findings on partner change, when incorporated into mathematical models of epidemic spread, is that any heterosexual epidemic of HIV infection in the UK is likely to be very slow-building.

Although the NATSSAL study did not collect time-trend data by follow-up study, it can nevertheless be used for time-trend analyses by comparing reports across different age-groups. These data show a tendency for multiple heterosexual partners to be increasing over time but they also show a sharp rise in condom use since the mid-1980s: less than 40 per cent of women who first experienced intercourse in 1985 used a condom, whereas more than 80 per cent of women first experiencing intercourse in 1991 used a condom (Johnson et al., 1994). Note however that these latter data illustrate time-trends but overstate the actual extent of condom use: condoms may often be used at the outset of a sexual relationship, but then they may be discarded as the relationship deepens (Kent et al., 1990). Unsafe sex in heterosexual relationships, as in homosexual relationships, may be associated with intimacy and trust.

A number of UK interview studies of young people have served to further explicate the low levels of condom use reported in heterosexual relationships. It is clear that knowledge of risk reduction practices is widespread: in a sample of 879 Glaswegian 18-year-olds asked what they understood by the phrase 'safer sex', 84 per cent mentioned condoms; among those reporting sexual intercourse in the last three months, the percentage was even higher (Macintyre and West, 1993). It is clear also that most young heterosexual respondents are more concerned about the risks of unwanted pregnancy than about the risks of

HIV infection (for example Health Education Authority, 1990) and that most respondents do not see themselves as vulnerable to infection, a perception associated with representations of the epidemic that ghettoise HIV infection into so-called 'risk groups' of gays and drug injectors (see, for example, Abrams et al., 1990).

As Wight (1994) has emphasised, the most striking characteristic of young people's sexual behaviour is its diversity. Among 16–24-year-olds in the NATSSAL study, 5.7 per cent had never had a sexual partner and 13.9 per cent had not had a sexual partner in the past year (Johnson et al., 1992). And many different studies have suggested that the commonest reported sexual relationship among young people is that of serial monogamy: among Wight's fifty-eight Glaswegian 19-year-old men, for example, a third were currently in heterosexual relationships that had lasted more than a year, with two respondents married, three engaged, and six living with the mother of their child (Wight, 1993). Most unprotected sex between young people occurs within these regular relationships. These unprotected sexual encounters are overlain with notions of romantic love, associating intercourse with intimacy, trust and self-sacrifice for the loved object. But the same encounters may equally (and simultaneously) be described by respondents in terms of a calculated understanding that one's partner is unlikely to be carrying a sexually transmitted disease.

The same romantic and calculative elements may be found in reports of unprotected sex with casual partners. Young women interviewed in Manchester and London for the WRAP (Women, Risk and AIDS Project) study were reluctant to describe themselves as having casual sex, hoping that their one-night stands would develop into steady relationships (Holland et al., 1991). And some of Wight's Glaswegian teenagers (Wight, 1993) would vary their condom use with casual partners according to their calculative perception of their partner: terms such as 'slag' and 'cow' have connotations beyond the abusive and controlling: they also serve to rank hierarchically perceptions of sexual risk.

However, heterosexual risk behaviour cannot be described adequately in ways which are gender blind. Women are at greater risk of infection than men. This is so because more heterosexual and bisexual men are already infected (particularly through syringe-sharing) than heterosexual and bisexual women and because the virus is thought to be more readily transmissible from men to women than vice versa. Yet despite their greater risk of infection, women are under more constraint than men in the adoption of self-protective strategies: in the negotiation of sexual behaviour women are restricted in their choices and may find themselves engaging in 'pressured', unprotected sex (Holland et al., 1992). The elements of this constraint are several.

Women have few leisure activities of their own, they are lower earners and less likely to be car owners: they may have more to lose than men from the ending of a relationship and their mobility at night is restricted. Male sexual desire is accounted as overmastering, with responsibility for controlling the Hyde-like transformations of her mate falling by default to the woman. But the carrying by women of condoms may be seen by others as polluting and indicative of promiscuity. There are double-binds here: women are supposed to be passive *and* to set the limits of sexual encounters; women are meant to be sexually attractive *and* forbidden to display and assert their sexuality.

Constraints on women's sexual behaviour may be conceptualised in Foucauldian terms: the sexual relationship is also a power relationship, a locus for the exercise of specific techniques of power and of resistance (Foucault, 1977, 1980). This is a topic that will be addressed more fully in Chapter 5, where different theories of risk behaviour are considered in detail. It can be noted here that, in addition to private heterosexual relationships, other social relationships involving risk practices can be considered Foucauldian 'strategic' relationships – private and commercial homosexual relationships, commercial heterosexual relationships and syringe-sharing relationships. But whereas in commercial sexual relationships, as was seen above, women may obtain directive control of the sexual encounter by dispelling the ambiguities that surround it, this strategy may not be open to women in private sexual encounters. In a revealing study of accounts of first experience of intercourse collected by Kent et al. (1990), many men and women reported that their first intercourse 'just happened', an unforeseen culmination of a mutely enacted series of events where ambiguity was both pervasive and functional. Ambiguity, undispelled by explicit communication, is functional in that it allows either party to withdraw without loss of face but it is also dysfunctional in that it allows accidental progression to risk behaviour.

Conclusion

If one were to identify a common thread running through these richly various sociological descriptions of HIV-related risk behaviour, it would be the situated rationality of those at risk. The practising clinician stresses health maintenance as a social task of overriding importance. This is a view to which others may pay lip-service but little honour: other tasks and other priorities may be more immediate. The continuing risk behaviour of those who know how the virus is transmitted is not irrational activity, a 'death wish' as Eric Rofes of the San Francisco Shanti Project and other (less well-informed) commentators have claimed. Rather, it may be seen as a rational response to immediate situations of risk – the exercising of strategic choices, deferral to strategic power, or the collaborative maintenance of a functional ambiguity.

The sociological and anthropological depiction (incomplete though it is) of this situated rationality is a considerable scientific achievement; it highlights the limitations of early policymaking on HIV prevention. Education is not enough. Provision of clean injecting equipment is a necessary, but not a sufficient, condition for the elimination of syringe-sharing. Where the social sciences have been less successful is in theorising about risk behaviour in ways which will suggest more effective preventive strategies. It is this theorising about risk behaviour which forms the topic of Chapter 5.

5

Theories of Risk Behaviour

There is a wide diversity of academic approaches to the study of risk, a diversity which stems not just from different disciplinary paradigms but also from different topical foci. Economists and engineers, for example, have attempted to forecast the probabilities of hazardous events, while lawyers have examined the control and regulation of risk. Among sociologists, interest in risk has concentrated on the topic of the various and conflicting discourses of risk. In part, this sociological preoccupation with public discourses of risk is a reflection of a wider political preoccupation with societal decisions about risks and, in particular, decisions about nuclear power (see, for example, the work of the influential German sociologist, Ulrich Beck, 1992, and also the recent Royal Society, 1992, review of risk analyses).

A similar interest in discourse analysis is to be found in sociological contributions to the field of occupational health and safety. For example, there are studies which explore the different and opposing discourses of risk used by unions and management (Hilgartner, 1985). Not surprisingly then, a similar approach can be found in many sociological studies of HIV/AIDS: Patton (1985), Treichler (1992), and Watney (1987) have all analysed the public discourses on HIV/AIDS in terms which reflect Foucault's earlier linking of discourses and power (Foucault, 1980). Public discourses on AIDS have been linked to public agendas for the policing of sexuality, the punishment of victims and the surveillance of deviants (immigrants, gays and junkies).

This Foucauldian approach to risk behaviour is heir to a long tradition of political commentary. As has already been mentioned, the same theme can be found in Daniel Defoe's *Journal of the Plague Year*, where he analyses the phenomenon of 'revenge infection' as a set of discursive practices (my terminology, not his!) mobilised by alarmed householders outside London to sanction their attempts to control and exclude the human tide of city refugees fleeing from the pestilence of 1666 (Defoe, 1986: 168). It is not rejection of this analytical tradition which leads me to follow a different approach in this chapter, but a different set of analytical concerns: the public health concerns that have sought to find explanations for variations in HIV-related risk behaviour as part of a strategy of epidemic prevention.

Social scientists' approaches to variations in risk behaviour may be sorted into three broad categories. Firstly, a social psychological approach with its intellectual antecedents in the theories of Kurt Lewin, which emphasises the role of variable perceptions (perceptions of vulnerability to infection, perceptions of the seriousness of the health threat, etc.) in explanations of risk behaviour – the 'health beliefs' model. Secondly, a cost/benefit approach which stresses the immediate rewards of risk behaviour (intimacy, the possibility of having children). And finally, a 'culture of risk' approach, first elaborated by the anthropologist Mary Douglas, which views variations in risk behaviours as stemming from different learned orientations to risk found in different sub-cultures.

Each approach will be examined in more detail, not just in terms of the illumination they provide on the reports of risk practices listed in the previous chapter, but also in respect of one particular study of risk behaviour – that conducted by the author on variations in risk behaviour among Glasgow male prostitutes. The male prostitution study is treated as a test case for the applicability of the different approaches. A brief report of this study precedes the discussion of the different theories of risk behaviour. The chapter ends with an overview of the deficiencies of each approach and suggests an alternative phenomenological approach with Schutz's work on 'systems of relevances' (essentially, a social theory of cognition) as a suitable heuristic scheme.

Risk behaviour among Glasgow male prostitutes

Fieldwork data were collected on thirty-two male prostitutes over a sixteen-month period. An attempt was made to estimate the size of the Glasgow male prostitute population over that same period (Bloor et al., 1991a), and the conclusion reached was that more than half the available male prostitute population in the city had been contacted.

Special efforts were made to minimise bias in recruitment of the sample. Street-working male prostitutes were recruited at a range of sites (two lavatories, two parks and two pubs) on a time-sampling basis. Recruitment did not proceed solely by introductions (the 'snowballing' method), but was also conducted by cold-contacting all observed prostitutes at the fieldwork sites. Male prostitution in Glasgow, as in other British provincial cities (see, for example, the report of Davies and Feldman, 1992, on Cardiff), is largely street prostitution. However, to ensure balance, off-street male prostitutes were also contacted through advertisements – escorts, masseurs and 'call-men' (prostitutes working from their own flats with 'books' of regular clients). More details of the methods of data collection and analysis may be found elsewhere (Bloor et al., 1992, 1993a).

Information on HIV-related risk practices was collected from all but six of the thirty-two respondents. Authorities such as the Terrence Higgins Trust have designated all ano-genital contact as unsafe because of the high rates of condom failure in anal sex, even for strengthened brands (de Vincenzi et al., 1991). By this definition, a significant minority of respondents (ten) were currently practising at least occasional unsafe sex with clients. These ten embraced a variety of biographical circumstances: they were off-street workers as well as street workers; they were gay-identified prostitutes and 'straights'; and they were novices and experienced prostitutes (including one respondent with four years' experience). The definition of *current* unsafe sex being used here is deliberately restrictive. A more inclusive definition might have embraced, in addition, one respondent who always sought to practise safer sex but had recently been raped by a client and also a second respondent who had only recently begun to work as a prostitute and had undertaken anal sex for the first time, but was resolved not to undertake it again as it was painful. Further, two respondents had practised anal sex earlier in their careers but were now unwilling to engage in it.

Yet even by this restrictive definition, unsafe ano-genital sex was being practised by a substantial minority of local male prostitutes. Other male prostitution studies, in the UK and elsewhere (Davies and Feldman, 1992; Morse et al., 1991), also report significant rates of risk behaviour. As we have seen, this is in contrast to female prostitution where studies throughout the developed world show very low rates of unsafe commercial sex.

However, comparisons between male and female prostitution may be misleading. Female prostitutes ensure that safer commercial sex is practised, often despite clients' preferences for unsafe sex, by maintaining directive control of the encounter from the outset ('Looking for business? It's ten quid for sex in a motor'). Male prostitution is a highly diverse phenomenon and, while some respondents pursued the same businesslike and directive approach as female street prostitutes, many others did not. Some respondents, for example, would mingle socially with their 'punters' (clients) in bars and discos, making no clear distinction between private and commercial sexual relationships. Similar ambiguities could be encountered at the lavatories and parks where prostitutes, like the respondent in my fieldnote below, often failed to make clear to their sexual contacts that payment was expected:

> He never asked for the money up front, although he remarked that he'd been minded to after he'd gone back to a punter's house and the punter had refused to pay. . . . He never even mentioned money afterwards unless the punter enquired about prices. He'd simply hold his hand out after the event and if he only got a fiver he'd say, 'Sorry mate, it's a tenner.' If the punter refused, he'd feign anger. Most then paid up.

The parks and lavatories were not primarily sites for commercial sex but for 'cruising' and 'cottaging' men who have non-commercial sex with men; the great majority of sexual contacts there were private, not commercial, encounters. Moreover, as was made clear in Humphreys's classic account (1970) of gay sexual encounters at American public lavatories, the stigmatised character of such encounters ensures that they are largely non-verbal. Thus, a degree of confusion between prostitute and private sexual traffic was frequent. But it should not be presumed that such confusion was inevitable: the respondent in my fieldnote below managed to make the commercial nature of the encounter evident at the outset. Indeed, his practice was not far removed from that of the female prostitutes working a few streets away:

> His procedure was to stand at the urinal. The client would come and stand beside him. When the coast was clear the client would put out a hand and he would immediately say, 'I'm sorry but I charge.' Some would leave at that point. With the remainder he'd negotiate a rate. He would accept £10 but sometimes got £20. . . . He always did handjobs or oral sex. . . . If clients asked him for anal sex he told them to eff off.

Comparision of those male prostitutes practising safer sex and those reporting unsafe commercial sex shows that unsafe sex was associated with client control. Not all punters were seeking unsafe sex, but those who were seeking ano-genital sex could only be deterred by prostitutes seizing the interactional initiative and openly discussing prices, type of sex and location.

One such means of seizing the initiative was to demand prior payment. Getting the money 'upfront' was the standard procedure among female street prostitutes but practised by only a minority of our respondents. Despite the fact that punters were resistant to prior payment (not least because they feared, with some justification, that the prostitute would 'do a runner' with the cash), these respondents reported that demanding prior payment was a viable strategy:

> I asked him if he took the money up front. He said he did and explained it had happened this way. The first time he got a customer he wasn't too sure how to proceed: the customer asked him how much he charged and he answered, 'how much will you pay?' Eventually they fixed a price. When they got to the venue he asked the customer for the money. The customer refused. So he said: 'No money, no deal.' And he got the money. He guessed from the customer's surprised reaction that it was more usual to ask for the money afterwards. But since he'd been successful he'd continued to work on this principle.

Getting the money first has the effect of opening up the 'hidden agenda' of the encounter, providing a conversational opportunity for the prostitute to make clear what he will and will not undertake at what price; it is strongly associated with safer sex. Seizing the interactional initiative, by this and other means, strips away the ambiguity that would otherwise surround the encounter. Without an interactional initiative from the prostitute, the punter's greater age might otherwise generate a natural authority in the encounter.

Thus, for the male prostitute, unsafe commercial sex is not a matter of volition based on perceived invulnerability to infection or similar perceptions; concern about possible HIV infection was widespread among our research subjects and only one respondent professed himself indifferent to the practice of safer sex. Instead, unsafe sex is associated with particular kinds of power relationships with clients:

> 'Simon' would do anal sex but *asked* [my emphasis] the punter to wear a condom. He also said, at a different point, that the punter was in control – things like type of sex and location were matters for the punter's discretion.

Unsafe sex is associated with client control. Safer sex is associated with countervailing prostitute strategies of power which dispel the ambiguities that surround the encounter and deny clients the interactional initiative.

In turning now to consider the different conceptualisations of risk behaviour in more detail, we shall also assess how far each different approach might provide an analytic basis for variations in risk behaviour among Glasgow's male prostitutes.

The 'health beliefs' model

The 'health beliefs' model (HBM) is one of several psychological approaches to the study of health behaviour. Others distinguished by Kronenfeld and Glik (1991) in their review of the field include the 'theory of reasoned action', 'social learning theory' and Weinstein's work on the 'precaution adoption process' (Weinstein, 1988). All these approaches conceive of risk behaviour as a volitional act and as arising out of the individual's perceptions or beliefs – the locus of the explanation lies with the individual rather than the group or the social situation. I shall deal solely with the HBM here, for simplicity's sake and because it is both the most popular psychological approach to health behaviour and the approach that has previously been applied to HIV-related risk behaviour – most notably in a Chicago interview study of a thousand gay men (Joseph et al., 1987).

The HBM derives originally from the theories of the social psychologist, Kurt Lewin, as Rosenstock, an early exponent of the approach has acknowledged (Rosenstock, 1974). It is argued that for individuals to engage in health behaviour, such as safer sex, an individual has to perceive him/herself as vulnerable or susceptible to a health threat, that health threat has to be perceived as having serious consequences, the protective action that is available has to be perceived as effective, and the benefits of that action have to be perceived as outweighing the perceived costs of the action. In fact, these variables have never had very much predictive power. In the above Chicago study there was only a modest association between perceptions of risk and the adoption of safer sexual practices. From the earliest days, exponents of the model have attempted to graft on more sociological variables. Thus Rosenstock, in an article modestly entitled 'Why people use health services' (Rosenstock, 1966), which attempted to explain both 'health behaviour' (the use of preventive health services) and 'illness behaviour' (the use of curative health services), expressed the view that even when individuals perceived that they could and should adopt a particular course of action, some trigger or cue might be required to nudge them into action. Elsewhere, the 'perceived costs' dimension of the model has been broadened to encompass perceived social constraints on the adoption of protective action, in recognition of the social structures and normative influences which shape and channel individual behaviour. Not surprisingly, in a review of the predictive performance of the HBM, Kronenfeld (1988) found that the 'perceived barriers to action' dimension was the most powerful predictor of health behaviour, ahead of 'perceived vulnerability' or 'perceived seriousness'.

The HBM is an improvement on rational economic models of decisionmaking, but for sociologists who see the wellsprings of action in the collectivity rather than the individual, these models of individuals' perceptions have little intuitive appeal. Rather than trying to graft collectivity-oriented dimensions on to individualistic models, it may be more logical to draw up new collectivity-oriented models, which treat perceptions as dependent rather than independent variables, shaped by social circumstances and situations.

These collectivity-oriented models have a long pedigree in the field of illness behaviour, where the psycho-social models of Rosenstock (1966) and Mechanic (1962) have been opposed by alternative conceptions which have stressed the structural barriers to the use of American health services and the need for such use to be culturally approved by family, friends and peers (see especially the work of Freidson, 1970, and Zola, 1973; also Suchman, 1965, Rainwater, 1968, and Strauss, 1969). A rough parallel, in the field of risk behaviour, to these sociological models of illness behaviour is found in the anthropologist Mary Douglas's work on risk behaviour (see p. 94 below).

Returning to the data on male prostitution, the difficulties are immediately apparent in conceiving of the Glasgow respondents' risk behaviour as volitional and shaped by, say, perceptions of invulnerability. Almost all those engaging in risk behaviour were very concerned about possible infection. Only one respondent could be said to be engaging in risk behaviour of his own volition:

> He never asked clients to wear a condom, if they wanted to wear a condom, that was their privilege. Very few did, he reckoned. How many of the clients he'd had in the last seven days had asked for straight [anal] sex? Four out of nine, he thought. How many had worn a condom? None. . . . He was perfectly aware of the risks of transmission but chose to ignore them. 'They're even saying that you can catch HIV from oral sex,' he said with a laugh. . . . He said he hated condoms, using them took the pleasure out of oral sex. . . . He wasn't interested in flavoured condoms either (said he might conceivably be tempted if they brought out a butterscotch flavour).

Other respondents practising unsafe sex were greatly concerned with the possibility of HIV transmission. Their continuing risk behaviour was not the consequence of a belief that the threat of HIV was small or that they personally were invulnerable. Quite the contrary. As we have seen, their risk behaviour stemmed from their inability to impose on clients their desire to practise only safer sex. A model of behaviour like the HBM, which conceives of risk behaviour as a volitional individual act, seems quite inappropriate for the analysis of behaviour which self-evidently involves two parties not one individual and which is characterised by constraint, not free choice.

The benefits of risk behaviour

An alternative approach has been to emphasise the situated rationality of risk behaviour by pointing to the contradictory social pressures on individuals and the immediate benefits that may accrue to risk-takers. This kind of approach is found in Luker's (1975) study of Californian women seeking repeated terminations. In her interviews she focused on the women's reasons for not using contraception and found her respondents providing numerous and diverse accounts for their lack of contraception. One woman believed that if she were pregnant this might galvanise her partner into defying his domineering parents. Another believed that her pregnancy might reduce the power her partner's ex-wife wielded through the children from that earlier relationship. Another cited the weight-gain she had previously experienced on the pill. In the situations Lukers describes reproductive decisionmaking may be influenced by a range of shifting and cross-cutting desiderata:

> In all heterosexual relationships (including those as brief as a single sexual encounter), people are trying to manage a number of complex tasks – only one of which is not getting pregnant – and they are doing so in a social and cultural context that puts contradictory demands on them. (1975 xi)

This approach has some affinities with social learning theory in psychology (Bandura, 1977) where emphasis is placed on the immediate incentives to risk-taking which may outweigh the more distant gratifications of abstention (for example, the immediate gratification of smoking versus the distant gratification of longevity).

A sociological study with a still closer affinity to Luker's work is Parsons's research on the reproductive behaviour of women at risk of bearing children with the genetic disorder, Duchenne muscular dystrophy: DMD (Parsons, 1990; Parsons and Atkinson, 1992). The variation in reproductive risk behaviour among Parsons's sample was not wholly explicable by reference to differences between the women in the risks they ran of bearing a boy with DMD: some women, advised by their clinicians that their child was at very low risk, would undergo amniocentesis and terminate a male foetus; other women, advised they were at higher risk, went ahead with their pregnancies. Such behaviour, which might be deemed irrational from a clinical perspective, was in fact the product of a situated rationality – a rationality with its roots in the women's social situations. For some women, the wish to form a family was paramount in their lives. For other women, their previous experience of growing up with a brother who had DMD may have been a positive or a negative experience, shaping their own family formation plans.

An approach to HIV-related risk behaviour which sees risk behaviour as the product of a situated rationality is implicit in many of the sociological studies reported in the previous chapter. Repeatedly, those engaging in risk behaviour in these studies have been reported as referring to the benefits of risk behaviour – the intimacy and trust between partners that is signalled by unprotected sex or needle-sharing, or the overriding wish of injecting drug users to have a family. Other respondents (like Wight's Glaswegian youths – Wight, 1993) have referred to a calculative appraisal that the risk of infection from their partner was remote and could safely be ignored. Yet other data suggest strongly that for some respondents the immediate gratification of an offered 'hit' outweighs the deferred gratification implied in the trip down the road to the distant pharmacy or the syringe-exchange. And similarly, immediate overmastering sexual desire or the excitement of the dangerous and forbidden may be accounted by heterosexual and homosexual respondents as reasons for engaging in unsafe sex.

There is much to commend in a sociology of HIV-related risk behaviour which treats such behaviour as rational and responsive to the risk-taker's immediate social situation. Indeed this is an old song in sociology. Many a student text whistles the tune of the necessity of understanding the social context in which behaviour takes place. And we all join in when W.I. Thomas's (1964) chorus-line is reached: 'If men define situations as real, they are real in their consequences.' Stressing the rationality of so-called deviant acts is a considerable advance on depicting them as irrational. Studies in the sociology of deviance, for example, have found considerable advantage in attempts to locate deviant acts in the local systems of meaning and sub-cultural normative practices with which those acts are associated. Macmillan's *Deviant Drivers* (Macmillan, 1975), for example, was an early attempt to apply this sociology of deviance approach to the topic of risk behaviour. However, the strengths of an approach which enables us to relate needle-sharing to specific aspects of drug culture, or to relate anal sex to gay pair-bonding, should not blind us to certain concomitant defects.

One such problem with the 'situated rationality' approach is the misleading implication of a calculative orientation to risk behaviour. The cost/benefit nexus is inescapably associated with models of economic rationality, with an open-minded weighing of the costs and benefits of various alternative courses of action. Economic models miss, of course, the social character of risk behaviour – the self-evident fact that unsafe sex involves more than one individual. But more than that, economic models miss the often unconsidered and frequently habitual character of risk behaviour. It is this aspect that a situated rationality approach is in danger of eliding. To emphasise the situated rationality of, say, needle-sharing is to combat the exasperated assumptions of irrationality, but it may also give a false impression of overly rational behaviour when the risk behaviour in question was merely unconsidered. The needle-sharing that may go on between sexual partners, for example, may be an habitual and taken-for-granted aspect of their daily lives, occurring several times a day without comment or reflection on costs or benefits.

To be sure, calculative risk behaviour does occur – the consideration among Glasgow youths that their prospective sexual partner is unlikely to be infected has already been instanced as one such calculative orientation. But a rounded approach to understanding risk behaviour would need to comprehend and emphasise habitual, as well as calculative, risk behaviour.

This leads us into a second difficulty with the 'situated rationality' approach. Most of the sociological studies described in the previous chapter are interview studies. As such, they perform a valuable service in giving a voice to the disadvantaged and the oppressed: the love that dared not speak its name can speak at last. But to privilege these respondent voices as authentic truth-tellers is to slip into a different project, that of the Romantic Movement, where authenticity is witnessed by the lack of distance between the speaker and the recorder of speech, where it is judged possible to break through veils of convention to the authentic 'inner self' of the research subject and to show that inner self to the world.

Interviewees, however, are not authentic truth-tellers artlessly revealing an inner self to the painstaking interviewer. Rather, interviewees are people being interviewed and their speech reflects the social situation of the interview. Some questions may have been asked of them before and their answers may have the rehearsed and fluent character described by Scott and Lyman (1968) as an 'account' and by Goffman (1968) as an 'apologia' or 'sad tale'. For example, many male prostitutes can give fluent accounts of how they drifted into prostitution (one of my respondents actually prefaced his biographical account with the words, 'Do you wanna hear a really sad story . . .?'), a fluency possibly born of previous conversations along similar lines with 'sugar daddies' and regular customers. Such practised accounts confound attempts by interviewers to pursue biographical topics like the possible association between childhood abuse and a subsequent prostitution career.

As serious as the practised character of interviewees' accounts is their natural bias against the adequate portrayal of habitual actions. Habitual actions are by definition unconsidered: in Schutz's (1970) analysis of routine activities the process of routinisation is simultaneously an erosion of reflectivity. And while an unconsidered routine can be reconstituted as problematic and reflectivity restored, this is no necessary consequence of the interview process and the interviewee may pass over unconsidered risk behaviour to dwell on those risks that have previously been cause for reflection. This leads us back to the over-calculative view of risk behaviour previously discussed.

Applying this 'benefits of risk behaviour' approach to male prostitution is no easy matter. The difficulty lies in the assumption that risk behaviour is volitional, that the prostitute may choose to risk infection for the benefits of unsafe sex. It is only if we use an extremely wide definition of 'benefits' that an application of the approach is possible – for example, we might see the benefits of prostitutes' unsafe sexual practices as the earning of income (assuming that there was no immediate market for safer sex) or the avoidance of intimidatory violence. The problem stems from our previous depiction of unsafe commercial sex as the product of client control of the encounter: the element of choice is present only for clients, not for the prostitute.

The conception of risk behaviour as a situated rational response thus ignores the fact that every sexual relationship (and every needle-sharing relationship) is a power relationship. Conceiving of risk behaviour as a volitional act only makes sense in respect of the dominant party in the relationship: in the case of unsafe commercial sex we may refer to the client's behaviour as volitional but not the male prostitute's. The point about power relationships applies more widely than the prostitute–client encounter: one party's choice is another party's constraint.

Power, according to Foucault (1980), cannot be wished or legislated away as if it were a commodity: it is inherent in relationships. The strategic character of the prostitute–client relationship is evident in the exercise of specific techniques of power. Safer commercial sex is practised by prostitutes who dispel the ambiguity that cloaks the encounter ('I'm sorry but I charge') and seize the interactional initiative ('No money, no deal') by the use of specific techniques of power. Unsafe commercial sex is practised by prostitutes who fail to contest the client domination of the encounter. Such passivity can hardly be characterised as the rational pursuit of the benefits of risk behaviour.

The culture of risk

The anthropologist Mary Douglas is the pre-eminent figure among those who see risk behaviour as a culturally variable product. In a series of publications through the 1980s (Douglas 1985, 1992; Douglas and Wildavsky, 1982) Douglas elaborated her 'grid-group' approach to risk behaviour and in 1990 explicitly applied this approach to HIV-related risk behaviour (Douglas and Calvez, 1990). Her argument is that variations in risk recognition, assessment and response are the product of local cultural variation – the product of differential socialisation in various sub-cultures and complex social institutions.

Variations in risk behaviour, it is argued, can be represented schematically by their placement in a two-by-two table whose two axes represent, respectively, the variable degree to which the individual is integrated into bounded groups ('group') and the variable degree to which those groups require adherence to particular rules of conduct ('grid'). In the resulting four-box table four different cultural orientations to risk (or 'cosmologies') can be distinguished: firstly, hierarchists (high grid and high group) whose risk behaviour may be high or low, in close conformity with the prevailing norms of their social group; secondly, sectarians or egalitarians (low grid and high group) who identify strongly with their own group, blame others for the emergence of hazards and are resistant to behaviour change; thirdly, fatalists (high grid and low group) who do not knowingly take risks but accept what is in store for them; and fourthly, individualists (low grid and low group) who stress the benefits of risk-taking.

A good example of the potential value of such grid-group analyses is Rayner's (1986) account of how responses to occupational radiation hazards varied systematically between different occupations in American hospitals. Rayner found that different hospital occupations' risk orientations could be classified according to the grid-group framework. Radiologists, for example, could be characterised as 'individualists' who viewed occupational radiogenic disorders (including some extreme case of fingers having to be amputated because of localised over-exposure) as a legitimate risk to be accepted in return for the humanitarian or material rewards of specialist medical practice. Similarly, maintenance workers such as plumbers, who had to clear 'hot' wastepipes through which radioactive materials had been disposed, could be characterised as 'fatalists', concerned about radiation risks but not operating in stable work groups and balking at collective or individual refusal to work with potential radiation hazards.

Douglas's own attempt to apply grid-group analysis to HIV-related risk behaviour (Douglas and Calvez, 1990) is less satisfactory. In particular, there appear to be difficulties with the differentiation of gay men from injecting drug users and the characterisation of injecting drug users as 'isolates' (or fatalists) with low group integration, a viewpoint which flies in the face of thirty years of ethnographic research on drug subcultures from Becker's pioneering study of marijuana-smokers onwards (Becker, 1953). Reports from large-scale studies of drug injectors have shown respondents to be following gay men in their dramatic reductions in risk behaviour (Frischer et al., 1992a) and ethnographic studies have shown that the disapprobation of casual needle-sharing in drug sub-cultures has similarities to the disapprobation of casual unsafe sex in gay subcultures. For example, this censorious report from one of McKeganey and Barnard's Glasgow respondents in the red light district:

> We asked three women we were speaking to if they were ever asked to lend needles and syringes. 'Oh aye, like that lassie the other night goin' round askin' everyone if they'll lend her a set. She even asked me but I said I don't carry any on me. I mean she asked me and I'm a stranger. She was askin' everyone, she could've used someone's that's got AIDS. (McKeganey and Barnard, 1992: 76)

Particular problems with the grid-group approach have been noted by Johnson (1987) and in the Royal Society review, notably the difficulty in allocating social groups unambiguously to one of the four basic cultural types. Indeed, some of the studies mentioned in the previous chapter would indicate considerable variability within social groups in their risk 'cosmologies'; differences within male prostitution would be a case in point. These difficulties may not be very serious. The grid-group approach may be conceived in terms of two cross-cutting continua rather than four discrete cosmologies, thus easing the placement of particular social groups. And the approach may be used as freely to analyse differences in cosmologies within social groups as between them.

More serious difficulties are raised by Bellaby (1990) who points to the static character of the model and its failure to account for the movement of individuals from one culture of risk to another. Bellaby suggests that a more dynamic and situated model is required, a suggestion that has affinities with the earlier analysis of male prostitutes' risk practices. In some instances the normative expectations and cosmologies that people bring to the situation of risk may be a less important determinant of risk behaviour than aspects of the situation itself. Risk-taking may follow less from learned orientations than from strategic relationships in the immediate risk situation. It was claimed earlier that the passivity of some male prostitutes who failed to contest client domination could not be characterised as the rational pursuit of the benefits of risk behaviour. Equally, to characterise such passivity as arising from a fatalistic cosmology is to understate the role of local power relationships.

Male prostitutes are a highly heterogeneous grouping: some of the Glasgow respondents were gay-identified and socialised extensively within the city's gay subculture, but others – including the drug injectors – did not gay-identify; some respondents mixed extensively with other prostitutes at the lavatories and other sites, while others were so isolated that they had never discussed their prostitution activities with anyone prior to their contact with the researchers. It might be supposed that the grid-group approach might explain the differences in risk behaviour between respondents in terms of differential group affiliation and relative autonomy from group control. Yet this is not the case. Those engaging in unsafe sex included both gay-identified respondents and others. And that group of prostitutes who hung around together at the lavatories followed no common norm of practice – even their minimum charges differed. Nor does the explanation lie in a distinction between novices and long-standing group members. While it is true that those who had practised as prostitutes for a longer period were more likely to be practising safer sex, some experienced prostitutes were engaging in unsafe sex and some novices (like the 'no money, no deal' respondent described earlier) had practised safer sex from the outset.

The Royal Society study group has rightly stressed the paradigm-shifting importance of the work of Douglas and her followers:

> The implications of this approach for risk assessment and perception are revolutionary. It implies that people select certain risks for attention to defend their preferred lifestyles and as a forensic resource to place blame on other groups. . . . That is, what societies choose to call risky is largely determined by social and cultural factors, not nature. (Royal Society, 1992: 112)

The grid-group dichotomy may be modified or rejected and a search may be conducted for an analytical framework which stresses the situated character of social action, but Douglas has made a lasting contribution in pointing to the cultural and institutional processes which selectively emphasise certain types of danger at the expense of others.

A phenomenological alternative

The phenomenological approach to a theory of social action focuses most strongly on behaviour that is unconsidered and on understandings that are taken for granted: the 'phenomenological attitude', so-called, entails the suspension of these unconsidered certitudes and an explicit analytical interest in the previously implicit. This social world of unconsidered certitudes and implicit understandings is the 'world of routine activities' (Schutz, 1970: 139), a world of familar topics, familar interpretations, habitual expectations, and automatic routine behaviour.

As was seen earlier, some risk behaviour may be calculative (for example, the considered view that there is only a remote possibility that one's prospective sexual partner is HIV-positive) but other risk activities (for example, regular needle-sharing and unsafe sex between a cohabiting couple) may be undertaken on a routine basis, without prior calculation or even any perception of the availability of alternative possible actions. This conceptual distinction, between two modes of cognition and social action, between on the one hand the social world of routine activities and on the other hand the world of considered alternatives and calculative action, is a central conceptual distinction in the work of Alfred Schutz (see especially Schutz, 1970 and Schutz and Luckmann, 1974). The same distinction between attention and habituation is echoed in many social science disciplines – in anthropology (Bourdieu, 1977) and at the confluence of psychology and neurophysiology (Mackworth, 1969).

In Schutz's work the distinction between attention and habituation follows a shift in cognitive practice that takes place when a person is faced repeatedly with the same stimuli. In novel situations, a person may consider various different interpretations of the phenomenon in question. Judgement may be suspended while the person inaugurates 'subsidiary projects' in order to arrive at a satisfactory interpretation; having arrived at an interpretation, the person may consider which among several associated 'recipes for action' should be embarked upon. Not all may be performable in the current situation and further subsidiary projects may be embarked upon in order to settle on a satisfactory recipe. But in the world of routine activities this elaborate cognitive process is collapsed, concertina-like: interpretation is no longer problematic but instantaneous and a matter of course; there is no distinction to be made between interpretation and recipe – the appropriate recipe for a given interpretation is a 'habitual possession' embarked upon automatically as an unthinking consequence of the perception of the phenomenon (Bloor, 1978). In one case cognition is a 'polythetic' (step-wise) process; in the other case cognition is 'monothetic' (a single flash). Theories of decisionmaking which treat all decisions as polythetic, as do those theories with their antecedents in economic costs/benefits, cannot be other than distorting. What is required instead is an approach which embraces the range of cognitive activity found along the novel/routine continuum.

Schutz's scheme of 'systems of relevances' is a heuristic device for the ordering of a range of cognitive activity within a single conceptual framework. It has been suggested (Bloor, 1970, 1985; Dingwall, 1976) that the range of activities subsumable under the term 'illness behaviour'(the perception of symptoms, their interpretation, the search for an appropriate remedy) might be conceptualised by reference to Schutz's scheme of systems of relevances. More recently, the same suggestion has been made in respect of risk behaviour (Bloor et al., 1992, 1993a; McKeganey and Barnard, 1992).

The systems of relevances refer to the varying ways in which we orient to perceptual stimuli: they are the bones of a social theory of cognition. Relevances are divisible into 'topical relevances', 'interpretative relevances', and 'motivational relevances'; each of these divisions is in turn sub-divisible, depending on whether relevance is volitional ('intrinsic') or constrained by others ('imposed'); and each set of relevances is of varying extension depending on two related but different factors – our interest in the project at hand and our degree of habituation to the stimuli. The scheme is represented diagrammatically in Figure 1.

Topical relevances determine whether or not a situation becomes problematic for the individual, whether or not interpretation of the situation becomes a topically relevant pursuit; intrinsic topical relevances refer to the voluntary pursuit of an interpretation, while imposed topical relevances refer to constraints. Interpretative relevances are the limited range of elements in the individual's stock of knowledge to which the situation in question may be compared. Assent to an interpretation will have different degrees of certitude – possibility, plausibility, probability; motivational relevances will determine how far the search for an interpretation is pursued, and the degree of certitude required. Once an interpretation is reached there may be a number of different 'recipes for action' attached to a given interpretation; further investigation may be required in order to ascertain which recipes are performable in the situation – constraints may apply to an individual's means as well as their ends.

This process of interpretation and action can be extremely elaborate: judgement on an interpretation can be suspended while subsidiary projects are embarked upon to eliminate alternative interpretations, or explore possible competing recipes. On the other hand, the process can be fleeting, both because of limited interest (motivational relevances)

Figure 1   *The sequence of cognition*

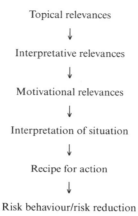

Topical relevances

↓

Interpretative relevances

↓

Motivational relevances

↓

Interpretation of situation

↓

Recipe for action

↓

Risk behaviour/risk reduction

and because of familiarity – the shift to a monothetic mode of cognition.

Schutz's scheme could be further developed (at the risk of trying the reader's patience!) but its heuristic value for the conceptualisation of risk behaviour should already be clear. Several advantages can be listed. Firstly, the focus is on the immediate situation of action, rather than on the orientations the individual brings to the risk situation. Secondly, Schutz's scheme can readily incorporate changes in risk behaviour over time as a consequence of shifting systems of relevances. And last but not least, the scheme embraces two dichotomies which we have previously seen to be pertinent to variations in risk behaviour and are unaddressed in the theories of risk behaviour discussed earlier – the polythetic/monothetic distinction and the volition/constraint distinction.

Turning back to the data on male prostitution, the variations in prostitutes' risk behaviours that were noted can be readily represented within Schutz's scheme. Thus, those prostitutes who reported current risk behaviour were not distinguished by group affiliation or perception of risk, but rather by the immediate circumstances of the sexual encounter: risk behaviour arose out of the immediate situation of action. Moreover, although for almost all the respondents avoidance of HIV infection was a topically relevant pursuit, many found their behaviour constrained by their clients. And those who avoided unsafe commercial sex did so by the adoption of certain strategies which enabled them to alter the strategic relationships with their clients: risk avoidance was a consequence of the adoption of certain performable recipes for action.

Conclusion

In the previous chapter, on empirical studies of variations in risk behaviour, some partial convergences could be noted among the rich diversity. Thus, although some reports have emphasised their research subjects' strategic choices in respect of risk behaviour (Hickson et al., 1992b; Wight, 1993), others reporting on needle-sharing in prisons (McKeganey and Barnard, 1992: 45) or on women's experiences of sexual risk (Holland et al., 1992) emphasised the way in which power relationships constrained risk behaviour: one party's volition may be another party's constraint. Likewise, a number of studies (Gold and Skinner's on Australian young gay men: 1992; Kent et al.'s accounts of first heterosexual intercourse: 1990) have emphasised the importance of immediate situational factors in the emergence of risk behaviour – the ambiguity of the situation, the lack of communication between the parties, and so on.

These affinities in diverse research reports could also be found in the risk behaviour of Glasgow male prostitutes but were not emphasised in the main theoretical approaches to the understanding of risk behaviour, particularly the 'health beliefs' model and Douglas's grid-group. One alternative approach has been to stress the situated rationality of risk behaviour and point to the contradictory social pressures on individuals and on the immediate benefits of risk-taking, but this approach brings other difficulties in its train, particularly when we consider risk activity which is unconsidered or habitual rather than calculative.

The diversity in HIV-related risk behaviour and the multiple deficiencies of coverage in the existing theoretical models suggest that attempts to move to a predictive model of risk behaviour may be premature. A more modest, but more readily achievable, goal would be a conceptual scheme in which these diversities can be described heuristically. Schutz's work on systems of relevance is one such possible heuristic framework. Schutz's analysis of the complex interplay of topical, interpretative and motivational relevances represents a series of cross-cutting continua where different ranges of risk phenomena may be located – from unconcern to militant determination, from inattention to weighted deliberation, from habituation to innovation, from the immediate to the culturally determined, and from the volitional to the constrained.

6
Conclusion

The aims here are, sequentially, to summarise the previous materials on the social transmission of HIV, to point to deficiencies and uncertainties in those materials, and to draw out some implications for HIV prevention policies.

Understanding the social transmission of HIV entails the location of the epidemic in its social context. The issues of concern and interest are not the biological mechanisms of transmission but rather the social relationships within which transmission occurs. I prefer to state the focus here to be 'social relationships' rather than the more conventional 'risk behaviour' because I wish to emphasise that transmission behaviour is not individual action but social action. It takes two (at least) to tango and all virus transmission occurs within particular and diverse social relationships – commercial relationships and private relationships, fleeting relationships and long-standing relationships, exploitative relationships and egalitarian relationships, and so on.

An early UK prevention campaign exhorted 'Don't Die of Ignorance'. In the later stages of the epidemic, when knowledge of the biology of transmission is substantial and widespread, the danger lies not in dying of ignorance, but in dying of (say) intimacy, or embarrassment, or powerlessness, or even ambiguity. These are complex matters, irreducible to simple formulas: as a campaign slogan, 'Don't Die of Ambiguity' has a limited potential. The task of a sociology of HIV transmission is to document and delineate the various and varying features of social relationships which amplify the risk of transmission. The task of health promotion in respect of the HIV epidemic is not to proscribe relationships, but to find effective ways to encourage modifications in those features of relationships which amplify HIV risk.

Trends in social transmission of HIV

The epidemic in the developing world
First, a warning. Summarising the previously reported material from Chapters 2 and 4 inevitably involves a degree of over-simplification as well as repetition: the African continent alone embraces much greater ethnic and cultural diversity than, say, Europe; and there are major dif-

ferences between the sub-Saharan African, the Latin American and the South Asian epidemics.

The character of the global HIV/AIDS epidemic is now transformed utterly from those early reports of immune deficiency in middle-class American gay males. The World Health Organisation estimates that, by the year 2000, 90 per cent of all AIDS cases will be in the developing world (Chin, 1991): it is now a disease of Third World poverty rather than First World affluence, with all that this implies for political commitment and resource allocation. Within the developing world, prevalence rates are highest in urban areas, but where the virus has spread among the rural peasantry it is rural poor (as measured by factors such as household possessions, type of house construction, land holdings and cattle ownership) who have the highest prevalence rates (Mulder et al., 1991).

The African epidemic is predominantly a heterosexual epidemic. Homosexual relationships are reportedly unknown or uncommon in many sub-Saharan cultures, although there is evidence that, in the past when the migrant miners of southern Africa were confined to the mining compounds and forbidden to visit women in the townships, 'mine marriages' between older and younger men were common; these mine marriages normally involved 'metsha' (a Xhosa term for rubbing the penis between the thighs) rather than anal penetration (Moodie, 1988). In Nigeria, injecting drug use associated with drug trafficking may be playing a significant role in HIV transmission. In the early years of the African epidemic contaminated blood transfusions and injection with unsterile needles (notably by traditional and lay healers) may have played a part in epidemic spread.

Our research knowledge of sexual behaviour in African societies is very limited. No national sexual surveys have been undertaken and local surveys may not have much applicability beyond the localities in which they are conducted, because of differences between tribal cultures and between urban and rural areas; anthropological studies emphasise this diversity of behaviour.

Epidemiological studies have stressed the central importance of female prostitution in the African epidemic. This is the 'core groups' hypothesis (Moses et al., 1991; Plummer et al., 1991). Developed initially in studies of the epidemiology of gonorrhoea (Yorke et al., 1978), the 'core groups' hypothesis posits a central epidemic role for female prostitutes as a consequence of their large numbers of sexual partners. The speed of the epidemic is only partly determined by the mean (average) rate of partner change in a population: it is also shaped by the variance around the mean – by the behaviour of minorities with very large numbers of sexual partners. Because the variance in sexual behaviour is very large, the behaviour of the minority having many partners may be more influential than the mean rate of sexual partnership in determining the rate of epidemic spread. Once HIV is introduced into a prostitute population, unless safer sex is being practised, the virus is spread rapidly between different prostitute women by clients patronising different women on different occasions; highly mobile clients, such as long-distance lorry drivers, transmit the virus between different local prostitute populations (Bwayo et al., 1992; Carswell et al., 1989). Infected clients in turn infect their wives and girlfriends. The epidemic role of prostitutes is said to be an important one, not just because of their large numbers of partners, but also because of the heterogeneity of their partners: their partners are not confined to a particular social circle, so that the virus is introduced into a range of different social groups (Plummer et al., 1991).

The 'core groups' hypothesis has been a source of some controversy, notably at the Amsterdam International AIDS Conference in 1992 where a morning session was devoted to papers on the topic. It was objected that the parallel being drawn between gonorrhoea and HIV may be an inappropriate one. In the case of gonorrhoea, the core is a self-sustaining source of repeated re-infection following repeated STD treatment. But, with no cure for HIV/AIDS, continuing replacement of dying core members is required. More importantly, gonorrhoea is much more readily transmissible than HIV, with transmission of the former occurring in approximately one in three exposures, while HIV transmission may only be occurring in one in every thousand exposures. This suggests that 'core groups' may only have an importance in HIV transmission similar to that in gonorrhoea when there is a high frequency of intercourse between members of the 'core group' and others, a pattern of behaviour not always found in prostitute–client contacts.

Anthropologists have pointed out that patterns of sexual mixing may vary radically between patrilineal and matrilineal societies: in the former, property is inherited through the male line of descent and women join their husbands' kin at marriage; in the latter, property is passed from the maternal uncle to the son and married women remain part of their family of origin (see Larson's 1989 review). Matrilineal societies are characterised by a degree of equality in sexual mixing. Comparatively speaking, in patrilineal societies divorce is uncommon and prostitution is common. Thus, although prostitution may play a prominent part in HIV transmission in some localities in Africa, such as Nairobi, where Plummer and his associates have been developing their 'core groups' hypothesis, prostitution may be much less prominent in other culturally contrasting localities, such as Kinshasa in Zaire. Even in Nairobi, different tribal and cultural groups practise quite different forms of prostitution, 'wazi wazi' and 'malaya'; the latter involves not just the sale of sex, but also the provision of food and lodg-ings, with quite different sexual mixing patterns from 'wazi wazi' prostitution (Day, 1988).

All these objections to the 'core groups' hypothesis may be met, but at the price of qualification of the hypothesis. Thus, novice prostitutes do indeed enter into prostitution, replacing AIDS victims. In Nairobi, the prevalence of HIV among prostitutes in a low-income area has remained around 80 per cent for several years, despite considerable population replacement (Moses et al., 1991). Moreover, the long latency period of HIV means that virus transmission by infected 'core group' members can occur over several years before sickness and death intervene. Again, although HIV may be inefficiently transmitted by single prostitute–client contacts, some types of prostitute–client rela-tionships involve frequent contacts and more efficient transmission: the 'malaya' prostitution practised by the Kikuyu women of Nairobi may be a case in point. And (perhaps most importantly) although, in gen-eral, HIV may be only inefficiently transmitted in single sexual contacts, the high prevalence of other STDs among prostitutes and their clients (particularly those diseases involving genital ulceration) will greatly increase transmissibility. Finally, although in principle the prevalence of prostitution may vary between patrilineal and matrilineal societies, population migration patterns have created massive local gen-der imbalances in many areas of Africa such that prostitution may be very widespread even in some traditionally matrilineal societies (Larson, 1989).

In sum, prostitution has indeed played an important role in the African epidemic, but the degree of that importance has varied from place to place, depending on local sexual mixing patterns, on local variations in prostitution practice, and possibly also on local varia-tions in the prevalence of other STDs. Prostitution also has a variable role in the Asian and Latin American epidemics.

Thailand and India are both countries with extremely large prosti-tute populations, sexual mixing patterns which favour rapid HIV spread, and relatively high prevalences of genital ulcerative diseases such as chancroid. Phongpaichit (1982) estimated the Thai female pros-titute population at half a million; Sittitrai et al. (1993) more conservatively estimate the population to be 150,000, with an addi-tional substantial number of male prostitutes. Although Thailand is well known as a sex tourism destination, the majority of the customers of Thai prostitutes are fellow Thais (Ford and Koetsawang, 1991). In a study of 2,417 Thai military recruits, 81.2 per cent reported past con-tact with a female prostitute and 57.3 per cent reported such contact within the past year (Celentano et al., 1993).

In both India and Thailand HIV infection among prostitute women has spread with extreme rapidity. In an overview of the Indian epidemic Shannuganaudan et al. (1994) cite increases in HIV prevalence among Bombay prostitutes from 1 per cent in 1986 to 38 per cent in 1994, and increases among prostitutes in Vellore, Tamilnadu, from 0.5 per cent in 1986 to 34.5 per cent in 1990. High prevalences among prostitutes are naturally associated with high prevalences among clients. In the previously mentioned study of recruits to the Thai military 12 per cent were HIV positive, but among that fraction who reported contacts with prostitutes weekly or more often, the HIV prevalence was 31.8 per cent (Celentano et al., 1993).

Injecting drug use may or may not have been an initiating factor in the Thai HIV epidemic. The very sudden 1988 explosion of HIV infection among Bangkok heroin injectors was discussed in Chapter 2. Female drug injectors are rarely encountered in Thailand and so a direct overlap between drug injection and female prostitution can be discounted, but early transmission from HIV-positive drug-injecting clients to prostitutes might be assumed, although the first known Thai AIDS cases were diagnosed in 1984, before the Bangkok drug injector epidemic (Ford and Koetsawang, 1991) and there is no molecular epidemiological evidence of a direct injector–prostitute transmission link. India too has experienced a sudden explosion of HIV among the drug injectors of Manipur in the north-east, abutting the Golden Triangle of opium production (Naik et al., 1991), but this may be merely coincidental with the growth of HIV prevalence among the (non-injecting) female prostitutes in southern Indian states such as Tamilnadu.

In Latin America there appears to have been a more limited epidemic role for female prostitution. Although the earliest AIDS deaths in Brazil were in 1983 and although levels of HIV prevalence of 11 and 12 per cent have been recorded among female prostitutes in São Paulo and Rio de Janeiro (cited in McKeganey, 1994), the rich erotic culture of Brazil (see Chapter 2) makes it likely that female prostitution will play a limited role in HIV transmission because female prostitute–client contacts constitute a comparatively small proportion of all sexual contacts – the ratio of the variance to the mean rate of partner change is reduced. Sexual mixing patterns in at least some Latin American states (Brazil included) are likely to show a greater degree of symmetry between males and females. It has been suggested that, although female prostitution is currently playing only a minor role in the Latin American epidemic, male prostitution could be of greater epidemic importance (Cespedes et al., 1992). Prevalence rates for HIV are high among some male prostitute populations (61 per cent in a sample of Rio street prostitutes: Van Buuren and Longo, 1991; 30 per cent in a Paraguayan study cited in Cespedes et al., 1992) and many of their male clients have regular and casual female partners. Outside the internationalised elites, Latin American cultures do not recognise the heterosexual/homosexual dichotomy found in Europe and America (and also in HIV epidemiology); instead they distinguish only between active and passive sexual roles and embrace a broad repertoire of sexual practices (Parker, 1987). Injecting drug use has also played an epidemic role in Brazil and Argentina, with an HIV prevalence among drug injectors in Rio matching, and in Santos exceeding, that found in Bangkok and New York (WHO Collaborative Study Group, 1993).

To reiterate the introductory qualifications, the developing world epidemic has been highly variable in its impact to date. Some African, Asian and Latin American countries remain only lightly affected: McKeganey (1994) cites HIV prevalence data from samples of female prostitutes reporting a nil prevalence (Sri Lanka) or prevalences of less than 1 per cent (Mexico). Nevertheless, in most developing countries where HIV has had an impact, prostitution appears to have played an unwitting role. The degree of importance of this role is locally variable as a consequence of differences in local sexual mixing patterns: in some cultures where women may take pre-marital and extra-marital partners, prostitution may assume less epidemiological importance; prostitution practice varies between cultures in the number and nature of prostitute–client contacts; and in some Latin American cultures it has been hypothesized that male, rather than female, prostitution has the more important (albeit still limited) epidemic role.

The identification of a pivotal role, if variable and imperfectly understood, for prostitution in the HIV epidemic has potentially grave consequences for groups of Third World women (and men) already vilified and discriminated against. But it is also an opportunity for the development of targeted services and improved conditions for prostitutes, since the practising of safer commercial sex could be both the main local bulwark against epidemic spread, and prostitutes' self-protection against sickness and death.

The reasons for limited condom use in commercial sex now have little to do with lack of access to condoms (although the work of Pickering et al. in the Gambia [1992] and Barnett and Blaikie in Uganda [1992] indicates that access to condoms may still be somewhat restricted in some rural areas). Instead, patterns of unsafe commercial sex are largely shaped by features of the prostitute–client relationship. Levels of knowledge of HIV transmission routes are generally high among samples of developing world prostitutes and most prostitutes are motivated to protect themselves by condom use (see, for example, Wong et al., 1994). Where unsafe commercial sex is occurring, it is in response to the wishes of clients, not prostitutes, and reflects the client's domination of the encounter.

The prostitute–client relationship is a 'strategic relationship' in the sense described by Foucault (1980), a locus for the exercise of specific techniques of power. Prostitutes may be disadvantaged by their economic dependence on clients, constrained by unsympathetic brothel owners, or cowed by intimidation or violence. Clients may be opposed to condom use because of unfamiliarity, or because of an anticipated loss of sensitivity, or because of a fear of loss of erection. The imposition of a condom may depend on the prostitute adopting specific countervailing techniques of power to seize the interactional initiative. This is a topic to which we shall return when considering prevention strategies (see p. 123). It is enough to note here that many studies of Third World prostitution show low levels of regular condom use (for example, the study by Nzila et al. [1991] of prostitutes in Kinshasa, Zaire, where only 15 per cent of prostitutes reported regular condom use with clients) and to note also that some similarly circumstanced prostitutes report more success than their sisters in negotiating condom use with clients: among 803 Singapore prostitutes, condom use was only successfully negotiated with about half of clients overall, but a minority of 30 women reported 100 per cent success in their negotiations (Wong et al., 1994).

The reluctance of prostitutes to use condoms with their private partners was noted in the discussion of Pickering et al.'s (1992) Gambian study in Chapter 4: the absence of the condom barrier signals a distinction between private and commercial partners and connotes intimacy and affection. However, where boyfriends live and work in the same social environment as the prostitute women (as was the case with the barworker boyfriends of many of the Gambian women), then the women are greatly at risk from their boyfriends, who can act as unwitting agents of cross-infection.

In this summary of trends in the Third World epidemic, we have focused on prostitution practice because of its pivotal epidemiological importance. However, much of the work on commercial sexual relationships remains salient in a consideration of private sexual relationships. Among the Ganda of Uganda, where prostitution exists but is of limited epidemiological importance and where there is rough symmetry in male/female sexual mixing patterns (Larson, 1989), many males are reluctant condom users. Masculine identity is associated with competitive sexual prowess and with fecundity (Barnett and Blaikie, 1992). There is little or no stigma attached to the contraction of a sexually transmitted disease. Women report interactional difficulties in introducing condom use into a sexual relationship, with their male partners believing that the suggestion signifies lack of trust or a belief that they are infected. Sexual relationships in developing countries obviously vary enormously in their strategic character, but in most instances latent economic power resides with men and privileges their sexual preferences; for women to impose condom use requires recourse to countervailing techniques of power. In the absence of such techniques, women may continue to practise unsafe sex even when they know their partner is HIV positive: in a sample of 138 Brazilian couples where the male partner had previously been diagnosed HIV positive, 17 per cent of the 75 couples still practising vaginal sex never used condoms (Castilho et al., 1991).

Men who have sex with men

There was a spectacular fall in reported risk behaviour among men who have sex with men in the mid-1980s. For example, in the San Francisco Men's Health Study already cited, the numbers of reports of receptive anal intercourse with two or more partners in the previous six months fell by 80 per cent between 1984 and 1987 (Winkelstein et al., 1988). This fall, which occurred across the developed world, pre-dated large-scale governmental campaigns and is attributable to self-help initiatives and major cultural changes within the gay community. Only a relatively small fraction of the change in behaviour is thought to be due to the removal from the community of the most sexually active through illness and death. This steep downward trend in unsafe sex in the mid-1980s was not sustained in the late 1980s and 1990s. There have been reports of increased HIV infections among homosexual men who had previously tested negative (Evans et al., 1993) and reports of increased male rectal gonorrhoea infections (Riley, 1991). Direct reports of the frequency of anal intercourse in cohort studies of gay men showed that a minority of men who had initially adopted safer sexual practices subsequently reported episodes of unprotected anal intercourse (Stall et al., 1990). However, there is no suggestion that levels of risk behaviour have returned to those levels found in the early 1980s. Overall, the cohort studies either found small continuing decreases in unprotected anal intercourse (Kippax et al., 1993), or no significant change in the numbers of penetrative partners (Hunt et al., 1991).

Of the various possible explanations for the recent apparent increase in reported risk behaviour among some men previously practising safer sex, the strongest candidate is that which points to an increasingly important role for type of relationship in determining risk behaviour. Most unsafe sex is reported with regular partners, while safer sex is normally practised with casual partners: unsafe sex is associated with intimacy, love and trust (Hickson et al., 1992a). This strategic decision to limit unsafe sex to one regular sexual relationship, often while both parties continue to practise safer sex with casual partners, has been termed 'negotiated safety' (Kippax et al., 1993); it involves an explicit or implicit negotiated agreement between the regular partners.

While anal sex between two HIV-negative mutually monogamous

men can hardly be designated 'unsafe', this is not the case for all sexual encounters between 'regular' partners. As previously reported, many gay men have more than one regular partner: 23.8 per cent of the UK's Project Sigma study respondents interviewed in 1990 had more than one regular partner and 4 per cent reported five or more regular partners (Hickson et al., 1992b). And those practising monogamy may be practising serial monogamy with a succession of regular partners; some regular partnerships may be of very short duration (Fitzpatrick et al., 1989). Thus an increasing tendency for gay men to discriminate, for self-protection, between types of relationship in the kind of sexual activity in which they will engage may have the paradoxical consequence of allowing some continuing epidemic spread.

A small minority of gay men are still engaging in unsafe sex with a large number of casual partners. In the 1987–88 Project Sigma interviews, 80 per cent of the sample reported ten or fewer male penetrative partners in the previous five years, but 4 per cent of respondents reported fifty or more male penetrative partners in the same period (Davies et al., 1990). Later data show reductions in numbers of penetrative partners, but still show a minority of respondents reporting multiple unsafe encounters: in a sample of 1,575 gay men recruited at the 1993 London Lesbian and Gay Pride March, 39 per cent of respondents reported that they had engaged in anal intercourse with a casual partner in the previous year, 9 per cent had engaged in *unprotected* anal intercourse with a casual partner in the previous year, and 3.5 per cent had engaged in unprotected anal intercourse with more than one casual partner (Weatherburn et al., 1994).

So one plausible epidemiological scenario is that of a small number of men with multiple casual penetrative partners acting as an epidemiological link between different networks of gay men where most, but not all, network members confine their unsafe sexual activities to one or more regular partners. This link seems feasible from published data: in the 1991–92 Project Sigma interviews, 29.1 per cent of men who had engaged in penetrative sex in the past year had engaged in insertive anal sex with both regular *and* casual partners, while 21.8 per cent had engaged in receptive anal sex with both regular *and* casual partners (Davies et al., 1993a).

This epidemiological scenario is, of course, a gay version of the 'core groups' hypothesis. A similar epidemiological role to that ascribed earlier to female prostitution might conceivably be ascribed here to male prostitution. Certainly, there are a number of studies of male prostitution, particularly in America but also in the UK and Continental Europe, which report high proportions of male prostitute samples engaging in anal intercourse with at least some of their clients (see the review by McKeganey, 1994). Davies and Feldman (1992) noted a tendency for anal sex to be more common with 'regular' clients than 'casual clients', but this was not a strong discriminator and 10 per cent of reported encounters with casual clients involved anal sex. Most commercial anal sex involves condom use, but rates of condom failure are higher for anal sex than vaginal sex. In comparision to female prostitutes, male prostitutes are less successful in maintaining directive control of the encounter with the client: matters such as type of sex and whether or not a condom is worn are often matters of client volition and unsafe male commercial sex is associated with client control of the encounter (Bloor et al., 1993a, 1993b). However, the epidemiological importance of male prostitution in the developed world can hardly be equated with that of female prostitution in the developing world, not least because of the large numbers of penetrative casual sexual encounters occurring outside of prostitute–client encounters. Data by Golombok et al. (1989) seem to suggest otherwise: in a postal questionnaire survey of 262 English gay men reporting a total of 3,778 anal penetrations involving different partners, 42 per cent were reported by just five respondents, all of them seemingly prostitutes. But there seems to be a sample bias here: it strains credulity to believe that, in a representative sample of gay men, one in fifty would be working as a prostitute.

Studies have been unsuccessful in distinguishing socio-demographically that fraction of men having same-gender sex who are practising unsafe sex. The relationship between age and unsafe sex found in some American data is not always apparent in data collected elsewhere. Respondents attending the 1993 London Lesbian and Gay Pride March showed no significant age differences in reports of anal intercourse (with regular or casual partners, protected or unprotected); analysis of data by length of sexual career (years since first sexual encounter) also yielded no significant differences (Davies et al., 1993b). American data also show higher frequencies of anal intercourse among non-white gay men, but it is unclear how far this apparent ethnic difference may be an artefact of unexamined differences in behaviour based on wealth and status.

There is similar conflicting evidence concerning supposed associations between practising unsafe sex and 'closeted' same-gender sex or bisexuality. American studies have associated the practising of safer sex with measures of acculturation into the gay community such as being a member of a gay organisation or regular reading of gay magazines or newspapers (for example, Seibt et al., 1994). In the UK, the recently published NATSSAL study is believed to have a much more 'closeted' sample than Project Sigma (which recruited from gay organisations), but the NATSSAL sample members reporting same-gender contact actually show lower proportions engaging in anal sex than the Sigma study (Johnson et al., 1994). American studies of men who have sex with men which report higher levels of risk behaviour for those who self-identify as heterosexual or bisexual (for example Doll et al., 1992) have not always been confirmed by studies elsewhere in the developed world (Boulton and Weatherburn 1990). Studies which seek to identify high-risk fractions of the population must be sensitive to their potential misuse for victim-blaming: Davies et al. deprecate those who would 'point the finger at groups marginalised not only by their sexuality but also from the established gay culture' (1993a: 175).

Some further difficulties should be briefly listed in depicting those men who have unsafe sex with men. Inadequate knowledge of HIV transmission is not associated with the practice of unsafe sex: all studies report very high levels of knowledge of HIV transmission. The 'health beliefs' model, developed to explain variations in health behaviour such as recourse to preventive dentistry, has been applied to HIV-related risk behaviour; it seeks to relate risk behaviour to differences in perception of risk – perceptions of vulnerability to health threat, perceptions of the severity of the health threat, perceptions of the efficacy of preventive action. The model has proved only a poor predictor of risk behaviour in a large American study of gay men (Joseph et al., 1987). The supposed association between intoxication and unsafe sex is absent from the Project Sigma data (Weatherburn et al., 1992); Australian studies showed no association between intoxication and unsafe sex, even when unsafe casual sexual encounters were considered separately (Gold et al., 1991, Gold and Skinner, 1992).

However, rather more successful attempts have been made to distinguish features of the immediate situation of the sexual encounter which are associated with safer or unsafe sex. The aforementioned study by Gold and Skinner (1992) of 15–21-year-old gay men showed an association between unsafe sex and a failure to communicate with one's partner about safer sex: where the ambiguity of the situation is not dispelled by explicit discussion, then the partner may be allowed to proceed by default to penetrative sex. The location of the encounter may be important. An ethnographic study of the sexual encounters that took place in the cabins of Stockholm's gay pornographic video clubs reported that very few cases of penetrative sex occurred because of the limited privacy the cabins afforded (Hendriksson and Mansson, 1992). Similarly, only a small proportion of sexual encounters in public lavatories ('cottages'), or at gay cruising grounds, involve penetrative sex (Keogh et al., 1992). Encounters at gay pubs and clubs are possibly more likely to involve penetrative sex because they are more likely to entail the parties' retiral to the privacy of a house or flat. In the Project Sigma data, those respondents who sought partners in public places went to 'cottages' frequently (a mean number of 7.0 times per month) but averaged just 1.6 penetrative cottaging partners per year; whereas bars were only visited a mean of 5.2 times per month, but resulted in 3.0 penetrative cruising partners per year (Davies et al., 1993a). In Amsterdam, where many gay bars have 'darkrooms' for sexual encounters, a similar fraction of gay men reported recent unprotected anal intercourse with casual partners in darkrooms (7 per cent) as in cruising areas (6.3 per cent) or gay baths (5.8 per cent); the same respondents were twice as likely to report unsafe sex with casual partners in private homes (13.3 per cent) – de Wit et al., 1994.

Although the gay community participated in an extraordinary public health achievement in the mid-1980s by their changes in risk behaviour, numbers of new cases of AIDS among gay men have continued to rise year after year, reflecting virus transmissions in the period prior to risk reduction. In England and Wales the number of new AIDS cases resulting from sex between men, adjusted for reporting delays, rose steadily from 182 cases in 1985 to 944 cases in 1991 (PHLS Working Group, 1993). At last, this rise is set to end (and has seemingly already ended in Scotland).

Injecting drug users
The spectacular fall in reported risk behaviour among men who have sex with men was mirrored by spectacular falls in reported syringe-sharing in studies of injecting drug users in the late 1980s and 1990s (for example, Frischer et al., 1992a). Stimson (1994a) estimates that current levels of syringe-sharing among UK injecting drug users are only a quarter or a third of those found prior to 1988. This public health achievement is all the more notable for having occurred among a section of the population who were thought by some to be unconcerned with, or inaccessible to, health education messages.

Most syringe-sharing that is still being reported occurs within very limited social circles – with a close friend, with one's regular sexual partner, or with a family member. Syringe-sharing, like unsafe sex, is found predominantly within particular types of social relationships and is emblematic of intimacy and trust (Bloor et al., 1994; McKeganey and Barnard, 1992). There have been some suggestions in the literature that the injection of certain drugs, such as amphetamines, or barbiturates such as Temazepam, is more likely to be associated with syringe-sharing (Klee et al., 1990a). This may depend on whether amphetamines and barbiturates are the only drugs injected, or whether they are part of a 'poly-drug' injecting career. In the case of those solely injecting amphetamines at least, the greater propensity to share on each occasion injected is likely to be more than outweighed by the greater infrequency, compared to opiates, with which amphetamines are typically injected (because they are not physiologically addictive): in a Glasgow study of 500 injectors the best predictor of reports of syringe-sharing in the previous six months was frequency of injection (Frischer et al., 1993). The same study also highlighted gender and lack of a fixed address as predictors of sharing. The greater propensity for female injectors to share may be because female injectors are more likely than male injectors to have a regular sexual partner who is also a drug injector – they therefore share with their sexual partner (McKeganey and Barnard, 1992). The greater propensity of those with no fixed address to share syringes may be indicative of a chaotic lifestyle, but it may also reflect the difficulty that a drug injector may face in refusing requests for drugs or injecting equipment from those to whom he/she is indebted for accommodation.

By no means all drug injectors in prison or on remand inject drugs while 'inside', but those that do so inject are much more likely to share, because of prisoners' lack of access to clean injecting equipment (Turnbull et al., 1990). Syringe-sharing in prison is of particular epidemiological importance because it mixes together drug injectors from different social networks, who may then transmit infection to their respective networks after discharge from prison. Residential drug treatment agencies may be playing a similar inadvertent transmission role to prisons, although this has not been systematically investigated (Bloor et al., 1989).

A syringe-sharing equivalent of the 'core groups' hypothesis has been suggested by Coleman and Curtis (1988) and more recently by Friedman et al. (1994), with a small group of injectors engaging in widespread sharing and acting as a transmission link between different networks of injectors. This is consistent with the known facts of the epidemic, but an alternative phrasing might be that transmission linkages between networks are made less by high-risk individuals than by injectors whose sharing patterns are shaped and constrained by particular adverse social situations, such as imprisonment or homelessness. HIV-related risk behaviour is not an individual activity; rather it arises out of particular social relationships and situational constraints.

In the early years of the epidemic, when access to clean needles and syringes was more difficult for drug injectors, then 'shooting galleries' (where injectors may congregate to inject newly bought drugs) and 'dealers' works' were important sources of infection. Shooting galleries are thought to have played a large part in the early American epidemic; dealers' works were thought to be implicated in the Edinburgh and Bangkok epidemics.

The phenomenon of 'drugs tourism' involves travel by drug users to obtain and consume drugs. It has been little researched but is thought to entail large volumes of drug users in some localities. For example, Arnhem, a Dutch border town of around 100,000 inhabitants attracts repeated visits (a mean of eight visits per year) from large numbers (500 to 800) German drug users (Grapendaal and Aidala, cited in Hendriks, 1991). Drug injectors who travel abroad in connection with their work or for holidays are naturally reluctant to carry clean injecting equipment through border checkpoints.

Sexual risk behaviour by HIV-positive drug injectors has long been recognised as an important route of heterosexual transmission of the virus. Of the cumulative total of 291 HIV and AIDS cases reports in England and Wales up to April 1993 involving heterosexual transmission with a 'high risk' partner, 159 (55 per cent) involved a partner who was an injecting drug user. In the US, more than 80 per cent of HIV-positive women either inject drugs or are the partners of people who do (Des Jarlais and Friedman, 1994). In the Edinburgh General Practice cohort of drug users where a 51 per cent prevalence of HIV was reported back in 1986, most new cases of HIV infection are resulting from sexual transmission, rather than syringe-sharing (Ronald et al., 1992).

It is a misconception that regular opiate users are not sexually active. In fact, the 500 drug injectors interviewed in the Glasgow study (reported earlier) and their counterparts in a parallel London study both reported a greater mean number of sexual partners in the previous six months (2.4 partners in London and 2.1 in Glasgow: Rhodes et al., 1993) than is the case for a comparable age-group in the UK NATSSAL study (Johnson et al., 1994). Once again, unsafe sex is associated with intimacy and trust: only 8 per cent of the Glasgow respondents reported always using condoms with their regular partner, whereas 16 per cent always used condoms with casual partners (Green et al., 1992). These low figures are probably broadly typical of the UK heterosexual population as a whole: only 23.2 per cent of men and 17.5 per cent of women reported using a condom on the occasion of their last heterosexual intercourse in the NATSSAL study (Johnson et al., 1994). Comparision of 1990 and 1991 Glasgow data shows a significant increase in condom use with casual partners, but not with regular partners: the 16 per cent reporting always using condoms with casual partners in 1990 had risen to 31 per cent in 1991 (Green et al., 1992).

There were 54 new cases of AIDS reported among injecting drug users in England and Wales in 1991. There were 27 such cases in Scotland, where new cases among drug injectors have outstripped those involving men who have sex with men. As Stimson (1994a) has pointed out, although these figures have been increasing year on year, they are far below earlier official projections. In 1988, the Department of Health was predicting 500 new cases per annum among English and Welsh drug injectors by 1990. Revised projections issued in 1990 estimated 400 such cases per annum in 1993. The 1993 Revised Day Report (PHLS Working Group, 1993) is now predicting 145 new cases of AIDS among English and Welsh drug injectors by 1997. There is thus the prospect of numbers of new AIDS cases starting to fall before the end of the century. But this will require not just the maintenance of current patterns of risk reduction among injectors, but also the absence of large-scale increases in drug-injecting.

The heterosexual epidemic in the developed world
In the earlier reading of the African epidemic, a crucial feature that distinguished the pace of the heterosexual epidemic in Africa from that in developed countries like the UK was the different pattern of female prostitution. In the UK the prevalence of STDs such as chancroid that cause genital ulceration is extremely low both in prostitute populations and in the wider population alike. There is also some evidence from male respondents in the NATSSAL survey of a long-term fall in UK client numbers, and only 1.8 per cent of male respondents reported paying for sex with a woman in the past five years (Johnson et al., 1994). But most importantly, all UK, European and American studies of female prostitutes and clients show that most commercial sex is safer sex (for example Day et al., 1988; European Working Group on HIV Infection in Female Prostitutes, 1993; Berry et al., 1992). HIV positivity among female prostitutes is associated with syringe-sharing, rather than unsafe commercial sex. Where unsafe sex does occur, it takes place despite the wishes of the women: unsafe commercial sex is associated with condom failure, with rape and intimidation, and with clients taking advantage of women's intoxication through drink or drugs (Barnard, 1992). Day and her colleagues (1988) have suggested that prostitute women are in more danger of HIV infection from their boyfriends (some of whom are drug injectors) than from their clients, since the absence of condom use in private sexual relationships is symbolically important to the women in distinguishing between private and commercial sexual encounters.

One possible qualification should be made to the claim that the health behaviour of prostitutes has proved one of the most important bulwarks against a Pattern II epidemic in the developed world. The qualification concerns the phenomenon of 'sex tourism', whereby developed world heterosexual and homosexual clients engage in unsafe commercial sex with prostitutes abroad, particularly in countries in the developing world. A Swiss telephone survey of men aged 17–45 reported that 1.2 per cent had paid for sex abroad in the previous nine months (Hausser et al., 1991). Thai police estimate around 100,000 male sex tourists come to Bangkok from the UK alone every year (Wilke and Kleiber, 1991). Noone et al. (1992) report seventeen known cases of HIV among UK travellers returning from Thailand in 1991 and 1992. An interview study with German-speaking sex tourists in Thailand reported that 46 per cent of respondents never wore condoms in their contacts with Thai women (Wilke and Kleiber, 1991). This greater propensity for unsafe sex in Thailand compared to prostitute encounters in Germany may be partly related to the power relationship between Third World prostitutes and sex tourists, which makes it more difficult for the women to insist on condom use. However, the researchers report that many respondents were reluctant to treat their relationships with Thai women as commercial, preferring to see them as 'holiday romances'. A parallel study of gay sex tourists in Bangkok reported less penetrative sex and more condom use in penetrative sexual encounters, but this was somewhat offset by respondents reporting more sex partners during their stay (Wilke and Kleiber, 1992).

Consideration of other aspects of heterosexual risk behaviour in the developed world has been facilitated by the publication of the results of various national sexual surveys such as the UK's NATSSAL survey (Johnson et al., 1994). The survey did not collect time-trend data on condom use but can nevertheless be used for this purpose by comparing reports on whether a condom was used at first intercourse across the different years at which first intercourse occurred. These data show a sharp rise in the use of condom at first intercourse since the mid-1980s, with less than 40 per cent of women using condoms at their first experience of intercourse in 1985 but more than 80 per cent of women using condoms at first experience of intercourse in 1991 (Johnson et al., 1994: Figure 4.8). Note however that, while these data are a good indication of time-trends, they greatly overstate the actual extent of condom use. Unsafe sex, again, is associated with intimacy and trust: condoms may be used at a first sexual encounter but as a relationship deepens condoms are often discarded. Only 25.9 per cent of women in the NATSSAL sample had used condoms in the past year; even in the youngest age-group (16–24) only 41.8 per cent of women had used a condom in the past year (Johnson et al., 1994: Table A10.1).

Low levels of condom use are not the result of inadequate knowledge of safer sexual practices (see, for example, Macintyre and West, 1993); most respondents in most surveys do not see themselves as vulnerable to infection, in line with media representations of the epidemic which associate virus transmission with so-called 'risk groups' of gays and injecting drug users. The most salient feature of sexual relationships is their diversity, but the most common form of sexual relationship among young people is serial monogamy (see, for example, Wight, 1993). Unprotected sex among young people is particularly associated with regular sexual relations and bound up with notions of intimacy and trust. Women are at greater risk of heterosexual transmission than men, but are also under greater social constraint than men, less able to adopt risk reduction strategies, and more likely to be pressured into unprotected sex (Holland et al., 1992). Sexual relationships are also power relationships.

The NATSSAL data on numbers of heterosexual partners indicated rather low rates of partner change. The mean number of heterosexual partners in the previous year was 1.2 for the men and 1.0 for the women (Johnson et al., 1992). Most epidemiological interest therefore attaches to that small minority of persons with large numbers of partners or high-risk partners. Although only a very small proportion of young people report high numbers of sexual partners, a high proportion of those reporting large numbers of partners are young people. A recent review of known STD cases among young people voiced particular concern at the relatively high rates of STDs in 16–19-year-old females, who had higher rates than their male counterparts and than older females (Clarke et al., 1993).

It is widely assumed that people are more prone to meet new partners while travelling than when at home. This assumption is only partially borne out in the NATSSAL study in respect of respondents whose work led them to stay overnight away from home: female respondents, but not male respondents, who worked away from home were more likely to report more sexual partners (Johnson et al., 1994). The picture is a complex one and it remains likely that certain kinds of travel experience are associated with partner change. The case of sex tourism has already been mentioned and some holidays are packaged to emphasise their 'romantic' connotations. The only national survey to ask specifically about partner change while travelling abroad was a Swiss telephone survey of 17–45-year-old men: 66 per cent had holidayed abroad in the previous nine months and 7 per cent had had a new sexual relationship with someone in the holiday country (Hausser et al., 1991). In a pilot study of a Nottingham general practice sample, 4.8 per cent of persons who had travelled abroad in the previous two years reported a new sexual partner on their last trip; men, single people and younger people were significantly more likely to report a new sexual partner (Gillies et al., 1992).

Some caveats need to be introduced here. Firstly, by no means all those encountering a new sexual partner while travelling are engaging in unsafe sex. In a study of out-patient travellers at the Hospital for Tropical Diseases in London, 54 per cent of those reporting a new partner never used condoms with that new partner; there was no tendency for condoms to be used less frequently abroad than with new partners in the UK (Hawkes et al., 1994). And secondly, meeting a new partner abroad should not imply that the new partner was a resident of the host country. A study of Swedish male travellers aged

19–21 years found that a third of their new holiday partners were Swedish women and a further third were tourists from other countries rather than women resident in the host country (Maardh and Kallings, 1990).

A study of nearly 2,000 Dutch ex-patriate workers returning from work in sub-Saharan Africa reported high levels of risk behaviour and five cases of HIV infection (Houweling and Coutinho, 1991b). A Belgian study of ex-patriates yielded similar findings (Bonneux et al., 1988).

Travel, transport and tourism workers can play an important role in HIV spread by providing links between local networks of sexual contacts. The possible role of long-distance lorry drivers in the African epidemic has already been noted. But lorry drivers are not the only transport workers who could be singled out for attention: cabin crews could also play an epidemic role and studies of seafarers show them to be between five and twenty times more likely than males in other occupations to contract gonorrhoea (Vuksanovic and Low, 1991).

Those working in tourist industries, such as bar and hotel staff, may also be vulnerable. In a study of migrant tourist industry workers in Torbay, Ford (1992) found that nearly half the male workers reported intercourse with four or more tourist partners; levels of condom use were only at a level comparable with the NATSSAL data; those reporting most partners also reported the lowest levels of condom use.

The 'Revised Day Report' (PHLS Working Group, 1993) on trends in the epidemic estimates that the proportion of HIV cases in England and Wales attributable to heterosexual exposure is currently a quarter of total HIV cases. It may be that this proportion will rise as a consequence of the gathering Third World epidemic. All developed countries can expect increasing numbers of HIV cases among migrants from developing world countries. This is a very sensitive topic with a strong potential for xenophobic public and organisational reactions. An EC report on HIV/AIDS prevention among migrant populations pointed out that the AIDS case data clearly indicate that, except in Belgium, the majority of current AIDS cases among foreigners in EC countries occur in other Europeans and Americans (Haour-Knipe, 1991). In America, although HIV is over-represented in the ethnic minority population, among immigrants the overall level of HIV infection is equivalent to that in the American-born population (Studemeister et al., 1990).

Uncertainties in the social transmission of HIV

Any attempt to summarise what is known about social transmission should address, not just the content of that knowledge, but also the degree of certitude of that knowledge. The planning of prevention interventions and services for persons with AIDS must embrace a range of epidemic scenarios and not just the likeliest scenario. Where considerable uncertainty exists, there is a need to plan for uncertainty. The wisdom of this is most evident in relation to the epidemic in developing countries, where even the most basic data on the epidemic are sometimes lacking. But it is also true of the epidemic in the Pattern I countries like the UK. In respect of the UK epidemic, uncertainties can be sub-divided into those concerning transmissibility, HIV prevalence, the prevalence of risk behaviours, and time-trends. There are also uncertainties concerning the effectiveness and efficiency of interventions, but discussion of these issues is postponed to the final section of this chapter.

It is known that HIV is much less readily transmissible than, say, gonorrhoea: James Chin, epidemiologist at WHO's Global Programme on AIDS, has suggested a mean transmission rate between 0.1 per cent and 1.0 per cent per exposure (Chin, 1991). It is also known that the virus is more readily transmitted from males to females than from females to males, that it is more readily transmitted via unprotected anal intercourse than via unprotected vaginal intercourse, and that it is more readily transmitted from insertor to receptor in anal sex than vice versa. But these differences in rates are very difficult to quantify. The difficulty is partly related to the sheer logistical problems of conducting research in this area: the most comprehensive study to date has been a collaborative European study which has followed up for four years 256 'discordant' heterosexual couples (that is, couples where one partner is HIV-positive and one negative); data were collected on more than 27,000 different episodes of intercourse (de Vincenzi, 1994); the mean transmission rate per exposure in unprotected intercourse was one per thousand exposures (95 per cent confidence interval: 0.5 to 1.7). But aside from the logistic difficulties, mean transmission rates by themselves may be misleading for a virus where we know that average transmission rates may be greatly enhanced by the presence of other cofactors, notably other STDs. There is an obvious association between enhanced HIV transmission and ulcerative genitalia due to a disease like chancroid; in one Nairobi study of GUM clinic attenders, 13 out of 113 women with genital ulceration became HIV positive over a period of just six months (Pattullo et al., 1992). But chancroid is rarely encountered in genito-urinary medicine clinics in the UK; more pertinent to the UK epidemic is a possible causal relationship with gonorrhoea. A causal relationship is difficult to establish because both HIV infection and gonorrhoea are independently associated with large numbers of sexual partners, but a causal association now looks very likely (see the review by Laga et al., 1991). In the European discordant couples study, seroconversion rates were significantly higher for those sexual partners reporting ulcerative genital infections *and* non-ulcerative genital infections (de Vincenzi, 1994).

Damage to the immune system also makes people with AIDS more susceptible to TB infection, but a reverse association also seems possible with TB leading to enhanced transmissibility of HIV.

Transmissibility is also known to vary with disease stage. Those who have AIDS (Stage IV disease) are known to transmit the virus more readily than those who remain asymptomatic; laboratory studies show that PWAs carry higher viral loads in their blood than asymptomatic patients. But it also seems likely that persons very recently infected are also more infectious in the weeks and months before they develop antibodies to the virus (Leigh Brown, 1992). This is one possible contributory reason for the seemingly characteristic epidemiological pattern of HIV infection among injecting drug users, where sudden explosions of infection have been recorded followed by a levelling out of HIV prevalence (see the discussion in Bloor et al., 1994). Transmissibility is also thought to vary between different strains of the virus and to vary according to genetic susceptibility, but studies in molecular epidemiology have shown that the main viral strains are widely geographically distributed and no study to date has linked genetic differences in susceptibility to infection with geographical differences in epidemic spread.

Turning from uncertainties in HIV transmission dynamics to uncertainties over HIV prevalence, uncertainties in the latter category are widely recognised because of the publicity given to successive downward revisions of offical projections of future HIV spread. Parenthetically, tabloid criticism of mismanaged official projections has been misplaced, because the estimates have always carried wide confidence intervals, and early estimates were based on very limited data, relying on back calculation from known AIDS cases. More recently, prevalence estimates and projections in the UK have been able to take into account data from unlinked anonymous HIV prevalence monitoring studies in antenatal clinics, neonatal blood testing, GUM clinics and drug treatment facilities (Gill, 1993), as well as data from the NATSSAL study. However, these additional data are themselves not free of uncertainties. Thus, the antenatal clinic data indicate only limited heterosexual transmission with very low proportions of HIV-positive women outside London and Edinburgh. But most women attending antenatal clinics are married or cohabiting and the NATSSAL data show that married women are significantly less likely to report recent multiple partners than those who are single (Johnson et al., 1994), so the antenatal clinic data may be understating HIV prevalence among women. Project Sigma data show an HIV prevalence fourfold higher for that fraction of the project's London sample who recently attended a GUM clinic compared to non-attenders (Hunt et al., 1992), suggesting that the anonymous testing programme in GUM clinics may be overstating HIV prevalence among men who have sex with men. The reverse has been the case in respect of injecting drug users, with most studies of drug injectors that have recruited samples outside of drug treatment agencies showing higher HIV prevalences than in agency samples, although this pattern may now be changing with large numbers of HIV-positive injectors attending drug treatment agencies for the issuing of oral methadone.

Controversy also surrounds attempts to estimate the size of the 'denominator' populations in these prevalence estimates – the proportion of the population comprised of men who have sex with men and of injecting drug users. In respect of the NATSSAL study, the authors believe that their proportions who report ever injecting non-prescribed drugs (0.8 per cent of men and 0.4 per cent of women) and their proportions who report injecting in the past five years (0.4 per cent of men and 0.3 per cent of women) are both likely to be underestimates, if only for sampling reasons – prisoners and those with no fixed address were not sampled (Wellings et al., 1994). The prevalences of same-gender sexual contact in the NATSSAL study (3.6 per cent of men reported previous genital contact with a man and 1.1 per cent reported a homosexual partner in the past year) were much lower than those in the volunteer sample of the 'Kinsey Report', but are 'remarkably consistent' (Wellings et al., 1994: 188) with other recent surveys conducted in France and Norway (Analyse des Comportements Sexuels en France, 1992; Sundet et al., 1988). The possibility of sampling bias can be excluded, but response rate biases may have occurred. The co-author of a comparable American survey, Charles Turner, has already been quoted on the likelihood of under-reporting (see Chapter 3). On the other hand, national sample surveys, relative to purposive samples of gay men recruited through gay organisations and the gay press, are likely to recruit higher proportions of men whose same-gender sexual activity is covert and 'closeted'; certainly the NATSSAL study shows a much higher proportion of men with same-gender sexual contact also reporting female partners, compared to reports of female contacts in the Project Sigma data (Weatherburn et al., 1992).

It is arguable that, in some respects, good information is still lacking on the nature and range of the risk behaviours whose prevalence is being estimated. This is certainly the case in relation to needle-sharing, where the permutations possible in sharing behaviour are numerous, but these different possibilities have not been set out systematically, let alone ranked in a hierarchy of transmissibility, or investigated for their relative frequency of occurrence. Research data are needed to produce a taxonomy of 'sharing', which would distinguish the various activities conventionally conflated under this umbrella term – the sharing of the needle, the sharing of the syringe, the sharing of both needle and syringe, the drawing of blood into the syringe to 'mix' a shared hit, immediate re-use of equipment, delayed re-use of equipment, and so on and so forth.

Some uncertainties over time-trends in risk behaviour have already been discussed in earlier chapters. The spectacular falls in risk behaviour that occurred in the gay community have not been partly reversed by 'relapse' into unsafe sex, as some American researchers have suggested. Instead of relapsing, some gay men have moved into 'negotiated safety' (Kippax et al., 1993), practising safer sex with casual partners and unsafe sex with partners of the same serostatus (see the argument in Davies, 1992 and in Hart et al., 1992). In a related way, some HIV-positive drug injectors have continued to share needles, but have protected their sharing partners from infection by always taking the last 'hit' from the syringe (McKeganey, 1990). Measures of changes in risk behaviours over time may not be particularly valuable if the social meanings of those behaviours also change over time: reports of continuing or rising rates of risk behaviour may be misleading if those behaviours connote with negotiated safety or 'safe' sharing at later points in time.

Uncertainties concerning time-trends exist, not just in relation to risk behaviour, but also in relation to some denominator populations. Particular problems are posed by possible changes over time in the size of the drug-injecting population. In the UK, time-trend data based on notifications of 'addicts' to the Home Office are suspect, due to widespread and fluctuating under-reporting. There were 142 notifications to the Home Office from the Greater Glasgow area in 1989, although at least 1,000 individuals were receiving treatment for drug use. In Glasgow it is currently possible to plot changes in the drug injector population over time, using 'mark-recapture' methods (Frischer et al., 1992b): the estimated 1989 population was 9,424 (Frischer et al., 1991). Extensions of this method offer perhaps the best prospect for accurately monitoring changes in drug-injecting populations.

Although researchers are unable to quantify the changes in drug-injecting that have occurred, it is widely recognised that considerable changes have occurred in the drug-injecting population and that the population is quite unstable. In the early 1980s there was a Europe-wide explosion of heroin use (Stimson, 1993), fuelled by imports of cheap brown heroin from Pakistan. In the UK, this population increase was concentrated in deprived urban areas. In some cities, such as Glasgow and Edinburgh, the heroin was injected from the outset, but in other cities such as Liverpool many users smoked heroin ('chasing the dragon'). Other urban areas such as South Wales were comparatively untouched by the epidemic. Instead, South Wales, in common with some other localities, experienced a later explosion of amphetamine injection, associated with a hepatitis epidemic (Clee and Hunter, 1987). Some existing heroin users became poly-drug injectors, injecting variously heroin, blackmarket prescribed opiates such as Temgesic (the drug of choice for Glasgow injectors), amphetamines, and barbiturates such as Temazepam. Some areas such as London and Bristol saw an increase in the use of smokable crack-cocaine, but other areas, waiting nervously for a crack epidemic that hardly materialised, were taken by surprise by rapid local upsurges in steroid injecting associated with body-building (Korkia and Stimson, 1993; Pates and Temple, 1992). In sum, the drug-injecting population has previously proved very unstable, future waves of injecting have not been predicted, and there has been limited overlap between successive waves of injectors – implying that the lessons of HIV risk reduction will have to repeatedly taught and learnt anew.

Implications for prevention

Interventions among injecting drug users
No prevention policies have caused more controversy than those collectively known as 'harm reduction' policies for drug injectors. The policies involve advice on safe injecting practice, better treatment facilities, substitute prescribing (particularly of oral methadone) and, most famously or notoriously, the provision of clean injecting equipment. There were 'Not-In-My-Backyard' demonstrations outside the new syringe-exchanges. Punches were thrown in a workshop session at the International AIDS Conference in Florence and the Italian police piled in to sort out the warring delegates. The policy is straightforward enough, suggesting that the dangers of HIV spread are a greater threat to the public health than the dangers of drug misuse and that policies to minimise syringe-sharing should therefore take precedence over the 'war on drugs'; those currently unable to abstain from drug-taking should be encouraged to inject safely. However, harm reduction policies clashed head-on with two influential movements: firstly, with 'Minnesota Model' drug treatment policies which stressed the encouragement of the ex-user's commitment to total abstinence (see, for example, Sugarman, 1974); and secondly, with 'moral majority' politicians and commentators who saw harm reduction policies as condoning drug use.

In parts of Europe the policy battle was quickly won. Amsterdam had begun syringe distribution schemes in 1984. In the UK, voluntary syringe distribution schemes started in 1986 and pharmacists began selling syringes; in 1987 government-supported pilot syringe-exchange schemes were set up at fifteen sites in England and Scotland. The schemes were evaluated (Stimson et al., 1988a, 1988b) and expanded; later, community pharmacy syringe-exchanges were set up and have proved particularly valuable in localities remote from the earlier exchanges. In America, opposition to syringe distribution was and is fierce and there are also legal obstacles to both distribution and sales. Some 'underground' syringe distribution systems were set up and harm reduction advocates undertook bleach distribution to facilitate sterilisation of injecting equipment. Some policymakers and government-funded researchers sat on the fence and pointed out that there had been no evaluations using 'gold standard' control trial methodology, but right up until 1992 no funding was provided for such evaluations (Des Jarlais and Friedman, 1994). American provision remains patchy.

Availability of clean injecting equipment is a necessary but not a sufficient condition for the avoidance of syringe-sharing. Since syringe-sharing is self-evidently a social rather than an individual activity, policy strategies for risk reduction must focus on interventions which aim to bring peer influence to bear on sharers. Sharing, as has been argued, occurs within strategic relationships. Changes in the culture of drug injectors will alter the constraints experienced by injectors in interaction with their fellow injectors and may modify the content of those strategic relationships. Outreach programmes in particular are likely to be more successful if they focus on the encouragement of changes in the drug-injecting community, rather than focusing on the individual injector (Rhodes and Stimson, forthcoming).

Some of the uncertainties listed earlier have particular implications for prevention policies. The instability of the drug-injecting population is a case in point. The public health achievement in reduced syringe-sharing is fragile, not because existing injectors are likely to revert in future to increased syringe-sharing, but because the drug-injecting population is unstable and subject to continual turnover. New injectors may move in quite different social circles to long-standing injectors so that the opportunities for diffusing a culture of harm reduction to new injectors may be limited: at one South Wales syringe-exchange steroid users asked if they could collect their syringes at a different time from other exchange attenders whom they regarded as 'addicts'. This implies that harm reduction services must not only remain in place, but must also have the inherent flexibility to identify and recruit new target populations of injectors. To simply service a long-standing and shrinking cohort of, say, attendant opiate injectors will not be enough; services must be able to identify, and deliver services to, populations of novice injectors. Clearly, good drugs outreach services are centrally important to HIV prevention (Rhodes et al., 1991; Rhodes and Stimson, forthcoming). Prison populations of injectors are of particular epidemiological importance. Syringe-distribution is an unpopular policy option in the prison service because syringes can be used as weapons. In the wake of the 1993 HIV epidemic within Glenochil Young Offenders Institution in Scotland, the Scottish Prison Service began distributing tablets for syringe sterilisation.

Oral methadone prescription is strongly advocated as a means of attracting drug users into drugs services, maintaining contact and facilitating the communication of harm reduction messages (Advisory Council on the Misuse of Drugs, 1993). It has frequently been used to maintain contact with and influence HIV-positive users. Stimson (forthcoming) suggests that there is too much plurality of practice in methadone prescribing, that more conformity with evaluated good practice is needed, and that current 'starvation' dosages typically prescribed in the UK have been set too low. Amphetamine injectors typically underuse drugs services relative to opiate injectors; there have been isolated attempts to prescribe amphetamines in order to attract more amphetamine users into drugs services.

HIV prevention among drug injectors represents good value for money. Basing his calculations on early UK predictions of 50,000 HIV-positive injectors by 1992 and contrasting this with current government estimates that there were only 2,800 such infections up to 1992, Stimson arrives at a cost per prevention of £716, in contrast to the current cost of AIDS treatment of £25,000 per patient (Stimson, 1994a).

Interventions in the developing world

For risk reduction to occur, there has to be a favourable social structural and social policy framework. Where this framework is lacking the HIV epidemic will continue to grow. Myanmar (Burma), one of the countries in the Golden Triangle of opium cultivation, is a case in point. The government was slow to recognise the HIV problem among its drug injectors and slow to disentangle HIV prevention policies from those policies aimed at discouraging opium cultivation and drug trafficking. The Myanmar government is not internationally popular and this has inhibited the development of international assistance with local HIV prevention. In the interim, HIV prevalence among drug injectors in some areas of the country has risen to levels unheard of elsewhere, levels of 80 and 95 per cent (Stimson, 1994b).

The earlier discussion concerning HIV transmissibility and the role of other STDs as co-factors has implications for intervention policies to combat heterosexual transmission in those developing countries where prevalences of STDs are high. It is argued that, since many common STDs can be screened for and treated, STD control programmes can run alongside condom campaigns and, by reducing the prevalence of STDs, HIV transmission can also be reduced. Such dual control programmes may be particularly effective when focused on vulnerable groups such as prostitutes. The World Health Organisation already supports such dual programmes. A two-year dual programme among prostitute women in Kinshasa, Zaire, reduced the proportion of new cases of HIV from 18 per cent per annum at the beginning of the study to 2.2 per cent per annum at the end (Tuliza et al., 1991).

Projects which seek to make prostitutes the agents of HIV prevention policy need to recognise the economic and social constraints under which the women work. In Thailand, this requires the collaboration of the bar and brothel owners to ensure that clients denied unprotected sex do not simply take their custom to more lax and accommodating establishments down the road (Ford and Koetsawang, 1991). Projects which seek to empower prostitutes to obtain the acquiescence of clients in condom use will be more effective if they involve prostitute groups in project planning and in the selection of locally successful strategies of countervailing power. A group of male castrati prostitutes in India resolved to seek an initial deposit from clients, thus placing themselves in a stronger position to insist subsequently on condom use. In a number of developing countries female prostitutes have acted as agents for condom distribution.

Targeted community interventions aimed at encouraging safer commercial sex are likely to be more effective than the so-called 'zero grazing' campaigns favoured by the governments of some developing countries, which seek to foster monogamy and pre-marital chastity. Certainly, the European experience has been that mass campaigns have been unsuccessful in reducing numbers of sexual partners, as opposed to increasing condom use (Wellings, 1992). Developing countries can least afford ineffective interventions, both because budgets are extremely limited and because large numbers of AIDS cases will impose crippling economic burdens while simultaneously reducing economic production. Ugandan central government expenditure on health in 1986 was just 64 cents per head per annum; even with funding added from the WHO's AIDS Control Programme, expenditure was only $2 per head (World Bank, 1987, cited in Barnett and Blaikie, 1992). Economies will have to grow rapidly to finance the costs of even very limited AIDS treatment and care at the same time as they are losing some of their most economically productive workers; for example in Tanzania coffee production (the country's most important export industry) has been seriously affected by the epidemic and Kenya has lost tourist earnings because of publicity in the West about the country's HIV epidemic (Barnett and Blaikie, 1992). AIDS is a development issue.

In the medium term, improvements in the relative economic power of women, particularly in increasing African women's access to land, should serve to alter sexual mixing patterns. But such changes in women's economic power would be vigorously resisted and, for some countries, medium-term solutions are already too late.

Interventions among men who have sex with men
As Shilts's (1987) social history of the epidemic has made clear, major changes in risk behaviour occurred among gay men *prior* to the development of governmental campaigns and interventions; these early changes can be traced to cultural changes and self-help organisations within the gay community. It is this potential for achieving risk reduction through cultural change that lies at the centre of one of the most successful documented intervention studies, the so-called 'gay hero' study conducted by Kelly and his colleagues (Kelly et al., 1991, 1992). In a controlled trial intervention embracing sixteen medium-sized US cities (eight intervention cities and eight controls), Kelly and his colleagues first of all used barmen in gay clubs and bars to identify those men who were the most popular members of the local gay scene. These popular gay men (around 10 per cent of the bar-using populations) were then approached and asked if they would be willing to act as 'gay heroes'; those recruited underwent an intensive group training programme focused particularly on techniques for intervening successfully in everyday social situations to convey safer sex messages to their gay peers. The trainees were committed to averaging an intervention a day and were asked to log all the interventions they attempted. Follow-up groups supported and reinforced the heroes' efforts. Measures of risk behaviour among bar patrons were collected immediately prior to, immediately after and some three months after the intervention. In the control cities, where conventional health education materials had simply been displayed in the bars, no change in risk behaviour was reported in the study period; in the intervention cities a 28 per cent reduction in unprotected anal intercourse was reported.

The gay hero study is consonant with much of the discussion concerning theories of risk behaviour in Chapter 5. The focus is on cultural change, not on individual change, intervention occurs in the situation of action rather than being removed in time and place, and risk behaviour is more likely to be a topic for consideration and action, rather than being habitual and unconsidered. Such intensive interventions are expensive in terms of set-up costs, but once cultural change has been initiated it may gather momentum, snowball-like, without the necessity for further input. Such intensive peer-influence interventions may thus be suitable for a range of target groups; indeed Kelly and his colleagues suggest that the approach could be adapted for use in developing countries. The central role of the peer group for adolescents also suggests them as a suitable target group.

But the 'gay hero' approach will not be suitable for all target groups. Among men who have sex with men, for example, the intervention would only be clearly successful among men who socialise with other gay men. A gay hero intervention is likely to meet with less success among those men in the closet whose relatively anonymous and fleeting same-gender sexual contacts are largely made in lavatories, parks, saunas and the like. Outreach work is likely to be more effective among the latter. Outreach workers visiting 'cottages' and 'cruising' sites would also be able to contact that fraction of the male prostitute population working at such sites. The MESMAC (Men who have Sex with Men – Action in the Community) Project, funded by the Health Education Authority and evaluated by Prout and Deverell (1994), embraced outreach work of this type.

Interventions to prevent heterosexual transmission

Sexual self-identification as gay, bisexual or heterosexual is a poor guide to sexual behaviour: men who self-identify as 'gay' may report sexual contacts with women and men who self-identify as 'straight' may report sexual contacts with men. Most studies of behaviourally bisexual men report higher rates of unprotected vaginal sex than unprotected same-gender anal sex (Boulton and Weatherburn, 1990). In a similar fashion, Stimson (1994a) has suggested that drug injectors have achieved more striking risk reductions in respect of syringe-sharing than they have in respect of unprotected sex, although some increases in condom use with casual partners have been reported. It may be that interventions designed to encourage clients to take self-protective measures against infection are likely to be more effective than those which encourage clients to take measures to protect their partners. But there are also other possible factors operating here, such as the fear that switching to safer penetrative sex with a female partner may lead to disclosure of covert sexual activity with male partners, or the disclosure of covert drug injection. Stimson has suggested that some drugs workers are embarrassed about discussing sexual matters proactively with drug injectors. Examples are not readily available of interventions which have suceeded in reducing bisexual risk behaviour and drug injectors' sexual risk behaviour.

Some couples (homosexual and heterosexual) with discordant HIV statuses may knowingly engage in unsafe sex because of the meaning this has for their relationship (Green, 1994). However, some sexual partners may acquiesce in unprotected sex because they are unaware of their partner's positive HIV status and it has been suggested that partner notification schemes may reduce such risk behaviour. Partner notification, also known as contact-tracing, has been a long-standing part of the treatment of STDs in the English-speaking world. It is less common in some continental countries like France. Partner notification can be by the infected person ('patient referral') or by the treatment and testing agency ('provider referral'); the latter is more effective (Landis et al., 1992). There has been some hesitancy about the implementation of provider-referral notification programmes for HIV. The main arguments against such programmes are three: firstly, the threat of violence from the partner towards the infected person; secondly, the difficulty of offering partner testing when tested persons are discriminated against by insurers and mortgage-lenders (a discrimination now removed in the UK); and, thirdly, the continuing lack of widely recognised effective treatment for asymptomatic HIV-positive persons, which denies the contact-tracer the possibility of offering any treatment benefit to a partner who tests positive. In the UK, these drawbacks have so far persuaded most (but not all) clinicians against provider-referral notification. In America the picture is less clear-cut, with some states having made partner notification mandatory, although many infected persons decline to nominate partners. In the pre-perestroika Soviet Union, 64 per cent of known HIV cases up to June 1991 were identified as a result of aggressive contact-tracing (Pokrovsky et al., 1991).

The relationship between HIV transmissibility and disease stage has possible implications for interventions which seek to reduce new infections by extending voluntary HIV testing schemes and/or by developing and extending partner notification programmes. (See, for example, the report of the partner notification scheme operating in the State of Utah – Pavia et al., 1993.) Such schemes are premised on the assumption that those who know that they are HIV-positive will reduce their risk behaviour. Although rigorous controlled trial data are lacking on the effectiveness of testing and counselling (see the review by Beardsell, 1993), a number of studies of HIV-positive persons do indeed contain reports by respondents of risk reduction (for example, Kelly et al., 1989; McKeganey, 1990). However, if infectiousness is greatest before HIV antibodies develop, then those engaging in risk reduction *after* testing positive will be engaging in risk reduction only after their period of greatest infectiousness has passed. This is not to deny the possibility that such schemes would cut infections, but the effect may be less than some proponents may wish.

The ability of female prostitutes to resist client pressure for unsafe commercial sex has already been documented. It is clearly essential for the restriction of the epidemic that these women continue to practise safer commercial sex and thus services need to be in place to support this. Professional outreach work is important here, not least in the supply of condoms. Good practice would involve professional outreach workers mobilising prostitutes as health promotion colleagues to carry safer sex messages to clients.

Relations between developing world prostitutes and developed world sex tourists represent a special case in their potential for heterosexual infection (Noone et al., 1992). But interventions may be most effective if targeted at the women and brothel and bar owners, rather than at sex tourists. Some travellers from the developed world have family links with the developing world; health promotion work with, for example, British South Asians travelling to the Indian sub-continent, needs to be undertaken collaboratively with a range of community organisations.

While schools represent the most convenient and economical sites for health promotion initiatives with adolescents, it is sometimes argued that schools-based work is perhaps least effective in reaching those most vulnerable, such as truanting adolescents. Schools-based peer-influence approaches may need to be complemented by alternative strategies, such as professional youth outreach projects targeted at the most vulnerable sub-groups of adolescents.

The heterosexual epidemic in the developed world is primarily an epidemic which impacts on women, but women are under more constraint than men in the adoption of safer sexual practices. This suggests that some health promotion interventions in schools, in the workplace, and at other accessible sites, could be targeted specifically at women, with a view to providing women with countervailing techniques of power to resist male pressures to have unsafe sex.

A US Congressional Staff Report stated succinctly the importance of sociology in the HIV/AIDS epidemic:

> A sociological perspective on AIDS is critical for research and policy because the transmission of HIV infection occurs through intimate social activities, successful intervention strategies are based on changing the behaviour of large groups of people, and effective treatment programs require detailed knowledge of the social worlds of persons with AIDS. (Albrecht, 1992: 1)

Some important work remains undone or incomplete and not all aspects of the sociological work that has been undertaken can be reported here: the emphasis on social transmission has precluded consideration of the treatment and illness experience of HIV-positive persons and persons with AIDS. Yet, as this book has attempted to document, much has been achieved, collaboratively and independently.

Celebration of that achievement is inappropriate while new cases of infection accumulate, and with the threat of further rapid epidemic spread in South Asia and elsewhere. But the achievement to date has been considerable.

References

Abrams, D., Abraham, C., Spears, R., Marks, D. (1990) 'AIDS invulnerability: relationships, sexual behaviour and attitudes among 16–19 year olds', in P. Aggleton, P. Davies and G. Hart (eds) *AIDS: Individual, Cultural and Policy Dimensions*. Lewes: Falmer.

Advisory Council on the Misuse of Drugs (1993) *AIDS and Drug Misuse: Update Report*. London: Department of Health.

AIDS Group of the United Kingdom Haemophilia Centres (1989) Seropositivity for HIV in UK haemophiliacs', *Proceedings and Transactions of Royal Society London*, B325: 179–183.

AIDS Letter (1992a) 'Criminal charges over HIV in French blood transfusions', 28: 5.

AIDS Letter (1992b) 'Screening of blood donations for HIV-1 antibody: 1985–1991', 28: 4.

Alan, D., Guinan, J. and McCalum, L. (1989) 'HIV seroprevalence and its implications for a transexual population', V International Conference on AIDS, Montreal [abstract W.D.P. 34].

Albrecht, G. (1992) *A Sociological Evaluation of our Experience with Aids: Research and Policy*. US Congressional Staff Report prepared for the American Sociological Association and the Spivak Foundation.

Analyse des Comportements Sexuels en France (1992) 'AIDS and sexual behaviour in France', *Nature*, 360: 407–400.

Ancelle-Park, R., Bletry, O., Baglin, A. et al. (1987) 'Long incubation period for HIV-2 infection' (letter), *Lancet*, 1: 688–689.

Anderson, R. (1989) 'Mathematical and statistical studies of the epidemiology of HIV', *AIDS*, 3: 333–346.

Anderson, R. and May, R. (1988) 'Epidemiological parameters of HIV transmission', *Nature*, 333: 514–519.

Anderson, R. and Medley, G. (1988) 'Epidemiology and HIV infection and AIDS: incubation and infection periods, survival and vertical transmission', *AIDS*, 2 (suppl. 1): S57–S63.

Bagasao, T., Quintos, M., Monzon, O., Giannone, P. and Asoy, L. (1990) 'Determinants of effective AIDS education and counselling among Filipino women at high risk of HIV infection'. Paper presented at VI International AIDS Conference, San Francisco [abstract Th.D.778].

Bandura, A. (1977) 'Towards a unifying theory of behavioural change', *Psychological Review*, 84: 191–215.

Barnard, M. (1992) 'Gender differences in HIV-related risk behaviour among a sample of Glasgow drug injectors'. PhD thesis, University of Glasgow.

Barnard, M. (1993) 'Violence and vulnerability: conditions of work for streetworking prostitutes', *Sociology of Health and Illness*, 15: 683–705.

Barnard, M., McKeganey, N. and Leyland, A. (1993) 'Risk behaviours among male clients of female prostitutes', *British Medical Journal*, 307: 361–362.

Barnett, T. and Blaikie, P. (1992) *AIDS in Africa: its Present and Future Impact*. London: Belhaven Press.

Bath, G., Burns, S., Davies, A. et al. (1993) 'HIV prevalence in injecting drug users, Edinburgh 1992'. Paper presented at *MRC AIDS Epidemiology Workshop*, Brighton [abstract 50].

Beardsell, S. (1993) 'Should wider HIV testing be encouraged on the groups of HIV prevention?' *AIDS Care*, 6: 5–19.

Beck, U. (1992) *Risk Society: towards a New Modernity*. London: Sage.

Becker, H. (1953) 'Becoming a marihuana user', *American Journal of Sociology*, 59: 235–242.

Beharrell, P. (1992) 'AIDS and the British press', in J. Eldridge (ed.) *Getting the Message*. London: Routledge.

Bellaby, P. (1990) 'To risk or not to risk? Uses and limitations of Mary Douglas on risk acceptability for understanding health and safety at work and road accidents', *Sociological Review*, 38: 465–483.

Berkelman, R., Fleming, P., Chu, S. and Hanson, D. (1991) 'Women and AIDS: the increasing role of heterosexual transmission in the United States'. Paper presented at VII International Conference on AIDS, Florence [abstract W.C. 102].

Barry, S., Kanouse, D., Duan, N. et al. (1992) 'Risky and non-risky sexual transactions with clients in a Los Angeles probability sample of female prostitutes'. Paper presented at VIII International Conference on AIDS, Amsterdam [abstract PoD 5604].

Bloor, M. (1970) 'Current explanatory models of pre-patient behaviour: a critique with some suggestions on further model development'. M.Litt. dissertation, University of Aberdeen.

Bloor, M. (1978) 'On the routinised nature of work in people-processing agencies', in A. Davies (ed.) *Relationships between Doctors and Patients*. Farnborough: Teakfield.

Bloor, M. (1985) 'Observations of abortive illness behaviour', *Urban Life*, 14: 300–316.

Bloor, M., Rahman, M., McKeganey, N. et al. (1989) 'Needle-sharing in residential drug treatment units' (letter), *British Journal of Addiction*, 84: 1547–1549.

Bloor, M., Finlay, A., Barnard, M. and McKeganey, N. (1991a) 'Male prostitution and risks of HIV infection in Glasgow: final report', *ANSWER*, A212: 1–3.

Bloor, M., Goldberg, D. and Emslie, J. (1991b) 'Ethnostatistics and the AIDS epidemic', *British Journal of Sociology*, 42: 131–138.

Bloor, M., Leyland, A., Barnard, M. and McKeganey, N. (1991c) 'Estimating hidden populations: a new method of calculating the prevalence of drug-injecting and non-injecting female street prostitution', *British Journal of Addiction*, 86: 1477–1483.

Bloor, M., McKeganey, N., Finlay, A. and Barnard, M. (1992) 'The inappropriateness of psycho-social models of risk behaviour to understanding HIV-related risk behaviour among Glasgow male prostitutes', *AIDS Care*, 4: 131–137.

Bloor, M., Barnard, M., Finlay, A. and McKeganey, N. (1993a) 'HIV-related risk practices among Glasgow male prostitutes: reframing concepts of risk behaviour', *Medical Anthropology Quarterly*, 7: 1–19.

Bloor, M., Frischer, M., Taylor, A. et al. (1994) 'Tideline and turn? possible reasons for the continuing low HIV prevalence among Glasgow's injecting drug users', *Sociological Review*, 42: 738–757.

Blower, S. (1991) 'Behaviour change and stabilisation of seroprevalence levels in communities of injecting drug users: correlation or causation' (letter), *Journal of Acquired Immune Deficiency Syndromes*, 4: 920–924.

Bonneux, L., van der Stuyft, P., Taelman, H. et al. (1988) 'Risk factors for infection with human immunodeficiency virus among European expatriates in Africa', *British Medical Journal*, 297: 581–584.

Boord, A. (1547) 'Breviary of Helthe', cited in M. Waugh (1989) Editorial, *Journal of the Royal Society of Medicine*, 82: 319–320.

Boulton, M. and Weatherburn, P. (1990) *Literature Review on Bisexuality and HIV Transmission*, Social and Behavioural Research Unit, Global Programme on AIDS. Geneva: WHO.

Bourdieu, P. (1977) *Outline of a Theory of Practice*. Cambridge: Cambridge University Press.

Brown, P. (1991) 'Why straight sex is not safe sex', *New Scientist*, 27 July: 17–18.

Buchbinder, S., Katz, M., Hessel, N. et al. (1994) 'Long-term HIV-1 infection without immunologic progression', *AIDS*, 8: 1123–1128.

Bwayo, J., Omari, M., Muteri, A. et al. (1992) 'HIV infection in long distance truck drivers: seroprevalence, seroincidence and risk factors'. Paper presented at VIII International Conference on AIDS, Amsterdam [abstract ThC 1514].

Cameron, W. (1990) 'Identification of biological cofactors in heterosexual transmission of HIV infection: epidemiologic observation and intervention in Nairobi, Kenya', in N. Alexander, H. Gabelnick and J. Spieler (eds) *Heterosexual Transmission of AIDS*. New York: Wiley-Liss, pp. 239–243.

Cameron, W., D'Costa, L., Ndinya-Achola, J. et al. (1988) 'Incidence and risk factors for female to male transmission of HIV'. Paper presented at IV International Conference on AIDS, Stockholm [abstract W.C. 45].

Campbell, C. (1990) 'Prostitution and AIDS', in D. Ostrow (ed.) *Behavioural Aspects of AIDS*. New York: Plenum, pp. 120–137.

Carrier, J.M. (1989) 'Sexual behaviour and the spread of AIDS in Mexico', *Medical Anthropology Quarterly*, 10: 129–142.

Carswell, J.W. (1987) 'HIV infection in healthy persons in Uganda', *AIDS*, 1: 223–227.

Carswell, J.W., Lloyd, G. and Howells, J. (1989) 'Prevalence of HIV-1 in east African lorry drivers', *AIDS*, 3: 759–761.

Castilho, E., Guimaraes, M., Sereno, A. et al. (1991) 'Condom use among female partners of HIV infected men, Rio de Janeiro, Brazil'. Paper presented at VII International Conference on AIDS, Florence [abstract M.D. 4060].

Celentano, D., Nelson, K., Suprasert, S. et al. (1993) 'Behavioural and sociodemographic risks for frequent visits to commercial sex workers among Northern Thai men', *AIDS*, 7: 1647–1652.

Centers for Disease Control (1987) 'Human immuno-deficiency virus infection in the United States: a review of current knowledge', *Morbidity and Mortality Weekly Report*, 36: S1–S6.

Cespedes, J., Easterbrook, P. and Quinn, T. (1992) 'Male prostitutes and heterosexual HIV-1 spread in Latin America'. Paper presented at VIII International Conference on AIDS, Amsterdam [abstract PoC 4039].

Chaisson, R., Moss, A., Onishis, R. et al. (1987) 'Human immuno-deficiency virus infection in heterosexual drug users in San Francisco', *American Journal of Public Health*, 131: 208–220.

Chief Medical Officer (1988) *Short-term Prediction of HIV Infection and AIDS in England and Wales* (Cox Report). London: HMSO.

Chin, J. (1988) 'HIV and international travel', in A. Fleming, M. Carballo, D. Fitzsimons et al. (eds) *The Global Impact of AIDS*. New York: Liss.

Chin, J. (1990) 'Current and future dimensions of the HIV/AIDS pandemic in women and children', *Lancet*, 2: 221–224.

Chin, J. (1991) 'Keynote address', VII International Conference on AIDS, Florence.

Chin, J. and Mann, J.M. (1988) 'Global patterns and prevalence of AIDS and HIV infection', *AIDS*, 2 (suppl.): S247–S252.

Choi, K., Kin, M., Catania, J. et al. (1991) 'First HIV seroprevalence survey in South Korea', VII International Conference on AIDS, Florence [abstract M.C. 3235].

Clarke, S., Gilbart, V., Noone, A. et al. (1993) 'HIV infection and other sexually transmitted diseases among adolescents in England', IX International Conference on AIDS, Berlin [abstract PO–C19–3059].

Clavel, F., Guetard, D., Brun-Vezinet, F. et al. (1986) 'Isolation of a new retrovirus from West African patients with AIDS', *Science*, 233: 343–346.

Clee, W. and Hunter, P. (1987) 'Hepatitis B in general practice: epidemiology, clinical and serological features and control', *British Medical Journal*, 295: 530–532.

Clumeck, N., Van de Perre, P., Carael, M. et al. (1985) 'Heterosexual promiscuity among African patients with AIDS' (letter), *New England Journal of Medicine*, 313: 182.

Coleman, R. and Curtis, D. (1988) 'Distribution of risk behaviour for HIV infection among intravenous drug users', *British Journal of Addiction*, 83: 1331–1334.

Cormack, R. (1989) 'Log-linear models for capture-recapture', *Biometrics*, 45: 395–413.

Coutinho, R., van Andel, R. and Rijksdijk, T. (1988) 'Role of male prostitutes in spread of sexually transmitted diseases and human immunodeficiency virus', *Genitourinary Medicine*, 64: 207–208.

Coxon, A. and Carballo, M. (1989) 'Editorial review. Research on AIDS: behavioural perspectives', *AIDS*, 3: 191–197.

Dada, A., Oyewole, F., Onofowokan, R. et al. (1993) 'Lagos Nigeria – New Dehli India HIV-1 connection among high class prostitutes'. Paper presented at IX International Conference on AIDS, Berlin [abstract PO–C07–2744].

Davies, P. (1989) 'Safer sex – still a long way to go', *Capital Gay*, 28 April.

Davies, P. (1992) 'On relapse: recidivism or rational response?', in P. Aggleton et al. (eds) *AIDS: Rights, Risk and Reason*. London: Falmer.

Davies, P. and Feldman, R. (1992) *Male Sex Workers in South Wales*, Project Sigma Working Paper No. 35. Colchester: University of Essex.

Davies, P., Hunt, A., Macourt, M. and Weatherburn, P. (1990) *Longitudinal Study of the Sexual Behaviour of Homosexual Males under the Impact of AIDS: a Final Report*. London: HMSO.

Davies, P., Weatherburn, P., Hunt, A. et al. (1992) 'The sexual behaviour of young gay men in England and Wales', *AIDS Care*, 4: 259–272.

Davies, P., Hickson, F., Weatherburn, P. and Hunt, A. (1993a) *Sex, Gay Men and AIDS*. London: Falmer.

Davies, P., Weatherburn, P., Hickson, F. and Keogh, P. (1993b) 'Risk of HIV infection in homosexual men' (letter), *British Medical Journal*, 307: 793.

Day, S. (1988) 'Prostitute women and AIDS: anthropology', *AIDS*, 2: 421–428.

Day, S., Ward, H. and Harris, J. (1988) 'Prostitute women and public health', *British Medical Journal*, 297: 1585.

De Vincenzi, I., Delmas, M., Brunet, J.-P. (1991) 'Prospective tests of nine brands of condoms by 319 volunteers'. Paper presented at VII International Conference on AIDS, Florence [abstract M.C. 3036].

Defoe, D. (1986) *A Journal of the Plague Year* (first published 1722). London: Penguin.

DeGruttola, V., Seage, G., Mayer, K. and Horsburgh, R. (1989) 'Infectiousness of HIV between male homosexual partners', *Journal of Clinical Epidemiology*, 42: 849–856.

Des Jarlais, D. and Friedman, S. (1994) 'AIDS and the use of injected drugs', *Scientific American*, 270: 56–62.

Des Jarlais, D., Choopanya, K., Wenston, J. et al. (1991) 'Risk reduction and stabilisation of HIV seroprevalence among drug injectors in New York City and Bangkok'. Paper presented at VII International Conference on AIDS, Florence [abstract M.C.1].

De Vincenzi, I. (1994) 'A longitudinal study of human immunodeficiency virus transmission by heterosexual partners', *New England Journal of Medicine*, 331: 341–346.

De Wit, J., de Vroome, E., van Griensven, G. and Sandfort, T. (1994) 'Safe and unsafe sexual intercourse among homosexual men with casual partners in different types of location'. Paper presented at Second International Conference on Biopsychosocial Aspects of HIV Infection, Brighton [abstract PO 35].

Dingwall, R. (1976) *Aspects of Illness*. Oxford: Martin Robertson.

Dingwall, R. (1993) 'Trouble at the Black Orchid: the ethnographic study of mass phenomena'. Paper presented at the BSA Medical Sociology Group Conference, York.

Doll, L., Petersen, L., White, C. et al. (1992) 'Homosexually and nonhomosexually identified men who have sex with men: a behavioural comparison', *Journal of Sex Research*, 29: 1–14.

Donoghoe, M., Dolan, K. and Stimson, G. (1991) 'Changes in injectors. HIV risk behaviour and syringe supply in UK 1987–90'. Paper presented at VII International Conference on AIDS, Florence [abstract Th.C. 45].

Douglas, M. (1985) *Risk Acceptability according to the Social Sciences*. New York: Russell Sage Foundation.

Douglas, M. (1992) *Risk and Blame*. London: Routledge.

Douglas, M. and Calvez, M. (1990) 'The self as risk taker: a cultural theory of contagion in relation to AIDS'. *Sociological Review*, 38: 445–464.

Douglas, M. and Wildavsky, A. (1982) *Risk and Culture: an Essay on the Selection of Technical and Environmental Dangers*. Berkeley: University of California Press.

Drucker, E. and Vermund, S. (1989) 'Estimating population prevalence of human immunodeficiency virus infection in urban areas with high rates of intravenous drug use: a model of the Bronx in 1988', *American Journal of Epidemiology*, 130: 133–142.

Duisberg, P. (1993) 'Can epidemiology determine whether drugs or HIV cause AIDS?' *AIDS Forschung*, 8: 627–635.

Easterbrook, P., Chiniel, J., Saah, A. et al. (1991) 'Factors determining racial/ethnic differences in HIV-1 seroprevalence in homosexual men'. Paper presented at VII International Conference on AIDS, Florence [abstract M.C. 3163].

Elifson, K., Boles, J. and Sweat, M. (1989) 'Risk factors for HIV infection among male prostitutes in Atlanta'. Paper presented at V International Conference on AIDS, Montreal [abstract W.A.P. 38].

Elifson, K., Boles, J., Sweat, M. et al. (1990) 'HIV-1 and STD infection among male transvestite prostitutes'. Paper presented at VI International Conference on AIDS, San Francisco [abstract F.C. 549].

Elifson, K., Boles, J. and Sweat, M. (1993) 'Risk factors associated with HIV infection among male prostitutes', *American Journal of Public Health*, 83: 79–83.

European Study Group on Heterosexual Transmission of HIV (1992) 'Comparison of female to male and male to female transmission of HIV in 563 stable couples', *British Medical Journal*, 304: 809–813.

European Working Group on HIV Infection in Female Prostitutes (1993) 'HIV infection in European female sex workers: epidemiological link with rise of petroleum based lubricants', *AIDS*, 7: 401–408.

Evans, B., McLean, K., Dawson, S. et al. (1989) 'Trends in sexual behaviour and risk factors for HIV infection among homosexual men 1984–1987', *British Medical Journal*, 298: 215–218.

Evans, B., Gill, N. and Gleave, S. (1990) 'HIV-2 in UK – a review', *Communicable Disease Report*, 1 (review no. 2): 3.

Evans, B., Gill, N., McGarrigle, C. and Macdonald, N. (1993) 'Sexually transmitted diseases and HIV infection among homosexual men', *British Medical Journal*, 306: 792.

Falciano, M., Ferri, F., Macedonio, A. et al. (1991) 'Heterosexual transmission of HIV: a four-year follow-up'. Paper presented at VII International Conference on AIDS, Florence [abstract M.C. 3070].

Faugier, J., Hayes, C., Butterworth, C. and Jeacock, J. (1993) 'Male clients of female prostitutes – risk behaviours and lifestyles'. Paper presented at IX International Conference on AIDS, Berlin [abstract PO–D10–3678].

Fay, R., Turner, C., Klassen, A. and Gagnon, J. (1989) 'Prevalence and patterns of same-gender sexual contact among men', *Science*, 243: 338–348.

Fitzpatrick, R., Boulton, M. and Hart, G. (1989) 'Gay men's sexual behaviour in response to AIDS', in P. Aggleton, G. Hart and P. Davies (eds) *AIDS, Social Representations, Social Practices*. Lewes: Falmer.

Ford, N. (1992) 'Safer sex in tourist resorts', *World Health Forum*, 13: 77–88.

Ford, N. and Koetsawang, S. (1991) 'The socio-cultural context of the transmission of HIV in Thailand', *Social Science and Medicine*, 33: 395–404.

Foucault, M. (1977) *Discipline and Punish: The Birth of the Prison*. London: Tavistock.

Foucault, M. (1980) *Power/Knowledge*, ed. C. Gordon. Brighton: Harvester.

Freidson, E. (1970) *Profession of Medicine*. New York: Dodds Mead.

Friedman, S., Neaigus, A., Jose, B. et al. (1994) 'Network and sociohistorical approaches to the HIV epidemic among drug injectors'. Plenary paper presented at Second International Conference on Biopsychosocial Aspects of HIV Infection, Brighton.

Frischer, M. (1992) 'Estimated prevalence of injecting drug use in Glasgow', *British Journal of Addiction*, 87: 235–243.

Frischer, M., Bloor, M., Finlay, A. et al. (1991) 'A new method of estimating the prevalence of injecting drug use in an urban population: results from a Scottish city', *International Journal of Epidemiology*, 20: 997–1000.

Frischer, M., Bloor, M., Goldberg, D., et al. (1992a) 'Reduction in needle-sharing among community-wide samples of injecting drug users', *International Journal of STD and AIDS*, 3: 288–290.

Frischer, M., Bloor, M., Goldberg, D. et al. (1992b) 'Mortality among injecting drug users: a critical appraisal', *Journal of Epidemiology and Community Health*, 47: 59–63.

Frischer, M., Green, S., Goldberg, D. et al. (1992c) 'Estimates of HIV infection in Glasgow from 1985 to 1990', *AIDS*, 6: 1371–1375.

Frischer, M., Haw, S., Bloor, M. et al. (1993) 'Modelling the behaviour and attributes of injecting drug users: a new approach to identifying HIV risk practices', *International Journal of the Addictions*, 28: 129–152.

Galli, M., Antinori, S., Esposito, R. et al. (1990) 'Seroseprevalence of HIV-1 among South American and Italian transvestites active in prostitution in Milan'. Paper presented at VI International Conference on AIDS, San Francisco [abstract F.C. 635].

Galli, M., Musicco, M., Gervasoni, C. et al. (1991) 'No evidence for a role of continuing intravenous drug injection in accelerating disease progression in HIV-1 positive subjects'. Paper presented at VII International Conference on AIDS, Florence [abstract Tu.C. 48].

Gellan, M. and Ison, C. (1986) 'Declining incidence of gonorrhoea in London. A response to fear of AIDS', *Lancet*, 2: 920.

Gephart, R. (1988) 'Ethnostatistics: qualitative foundations for quantitative research', *Qualitative Research Methods*, no. 12. Newbury Park: Sage.

Gill, N. (1993) 'Unlinked anonymous monitoring of HIV prevalence in England and Wales: 1990–92'. Paper presented at MRC AIDS Programme Workshop. Brighton: University of Sussex.

Gill, N., Adler, M. and Day, N. (1989) 'Monitoring the prevalence of HIV', *British Medical Journal*, 299: 1295–1298.

Gill, N., Heptonstall, J. and Porter, K. (1991) 'Occupational transmission of HIV', unpublished ms. London: PHLS Communicable Disease Surveillance Centre.

Gillies, P., Slack, R., Stoddart, N. and Conway S. (1992) 'HIV-related risk behaviour in UK holiday-makers', *AIDS*, 6: 339–342.

Goedert, J., Eyster, M., Biggar, R. and Blattner, W. (1987) 'Heterosexual transmission of human immunodeficiency virus', *Journal of American Medical Association*, 258: 788–790.

Goffman, E. (1968) *Asylums*. Harmondsworth: Penguin.

Gold, R. and Skinner, M. (1992) 'Situational factors and thought processes associated with unprotected intercourse in young gay men', *AIDS*, 6: 1021–1030.

Gold, R., Skinner, M., Grant, P. and Plummer, D. (1991) 'Situational factors and thought processes associated with unprotected intercourse in gay men', *Psychology and Health*, 5: 259–278.

Goldberg, D., MacKinnon, H., Smith, R. et al. (1992) 'Prevalence of human immunodeficiency virus among childbearing women and those undergoing termination of pregnancy: multidisciplinary steering group study', *British Medical Journal*, 304: 1082–1085.

Golden, E., Fullilove, M., Fullilove, R. et al. (1990) 'The effects of gender and crack use on high risk behaviours'. Paper presented at VI International Conference on AIDS, San Francisco [abstract F.C. 742].

Golombok, S., Sketchley, J. and Rust, S. (1989) 'Condom use among homosexual men', *AIDS Care*, 1: 27–34.

Gottlieb, M. et al. (1981) 'Pneumocystis pneumonia – Los Angeles', *Morbidity and Mortality Weekly*, 30: 250–252.

Green, G. (1994) 'Sex, love and HIV: the impact of an HIV-positive diagnosis upon the sexual relationships of men and women with HIV'. Paper presented at British Sociological Association Annual Conference, Preston.

Green, S., Taylor, A., Bloor, M. and McKeganey, N. (1992) 'Selective increase in condom usage among drug injectors in Glasgow'. Paper presented at VIII International Conference on AIDS, Amsterdam [abstract PoD 5382].

Guertler, L., Liomba, N.G., Eberle, J., Ntaba, H.M. et al. (1989) 'Comparison of the age distribution of anti HIV-1 and anti HBC in an urban population from Malawi'. Paper presented at V International Conference on AIDS, Montreal.

Handsfield, H. (1989) 'Trends in gonorrhoea in homosexually active men in King County Washington 1989', *Morbidity and Mortality Weekly Report*, 38: 762–764.

Haour-Knipe, M. (1991) *EC-Concerted Action on Assessment of AIDS/HIV Prevention Strategies, Migrants and Travellers Group: Final Report*. Lausanne: Institut Universitaire de Médecine Sociale et Preventive.

Harris, N., Sohlberg, E. and Livingstone, G. (1990) 'HIV spread among intravenous drug users in King County, Washington'. Paper presented at VI International Conference on AIDS, San Francisco [abstract F.C. 564].

Hart, G., Boulton, M., Fitzpatrick, R. et al. (1992) '"Relapse" to unsafe sexual behaviour among gay men: a critique of recent behavioural HIV/AIDS research', *Sociology of Health and Illness*, 14: 216–232.

Hartnoll, R., Daviand, E., Lewis, R. and Mitcheson, M. (1985) *Drug Problems: Assessing Local Needs*. London: Birkbeck College, Drug Indicators Project.

Hausser, D., Zimmerman, E., Dubois-Arber, F. and Paccaud, F. (1991) *Evaluation of the AIDS Prevention Strategy in Switzerland. Third Assessment Report (1989–1990)*. Lausanne: Institut Universitaire de Médecine Sociale et Preventive.

Haw, S., Frischer, M., Donoghoe, M. et al. (1992) 'The importance of multi-site sampling in determining the prevalence of HIV among drug injectors in Glasgow and London' (letter), *AIDS*, 6: 11–12.

Hawkes, S., Hart, G., Johnson, A. et al. (1994) 'Risk behaviour and HIV prevalence in international travellers', *AIDS*, 8: 247–252.

Hayes, R. (1991) 'STD Interactions – implications for control'. Paper presented at MRC AIDS Epidemiology Workshop, Brighton: University of Sussex.

Hays, R., Kegeles, S. and Coates, T. (1992) 'Changes in peer norms and sexual enjoyment predict changes in sexual risk-taking among young gay men'. Paper presented at VIII International Conference on AIDS, Amsterdam [abstract PoD 5183].

Health Education Authority (1990) *Young Adults' Health and Lifestyle: Sexual Behaviour*. London: HEA.

Hendriks, A. (1991) *AIDS and Mobility. The Impact of International Mobility on the Spread of HIV and the Need and Possibility for AIDS/HIV Prevention Programmes*. Copenhagen: Regional Office for Europe of the World Health Organisation.

Hendriksson, B. and Mansson, S. (1992) 'Sexual negotiations: an ethnographic study of men who have sex with men'. Paper presented at VIII International Conference on AIDS, Amsterdam [abstract PoD 5184].

Hickson, F., Weatherburn, P., Davies, P. et al. (1992a) 'Why gay men engage in anal intercourse'. Paper presented at VIII International Conference on AIDS, Amsterdam [abstract PoD 5185].

Hickson, F., Davies, P., Hunt, A. et al. (1992b) 'Maintenance of open gay relationships: some strategies for protection against HIV', *AIDS Care*, 4: 409–419.

Hickson, F., Davies, P., Hunt, A. et al. (1994) 'Gay men as victims of non-consensual sex', *Archives of Sexual Behaviour*, 23: 1–15.

Hilgartner, S. (1985) 'The political language of risk, defining occupational health', in D. Nelkin (ed.) *The Language of Risk*. London: Sage.

Ho, D., Neumann, A., Perelson, A. et al. (1995) 'Rapid turnover of plasma virions and CD4 lymphocytes in HIV-1 infection', *Nature*, 373: 123–126.

Holland, J., Ramazanoglu, C., Scott, S., Sharpe, S. and Thomson, R. (1991) 'Sex, gender and power: young women's sexuality in the shadow of AIDS', *Sociology of Health and Illness*, 12: 336–350.

Holland, J., Ramazanoglu, C., Sharpe, S. and Thompson, R. (1992) 'Pressured pleasure: young women and the negotiation of sexual boundaries', *Sociological Review*, 40: 645–674.

Houweling, H. and Coutinho, R. (1991a) 'Acquired immune deficiency syndrome (AIDS)', in W. Holland et al. (eds) *Oxford Textbook of Public Health*, Oxford: Oxford University Press.

Houweling, H. and Coutinho, R. (1991b) 'Risk of HIV infection among Dutch expatriates in Sub-Saharan Africa', *International Journal of STD and AIDS*, 2: 252–257.

Howard, J. and Borges, P. (1970) 'Needle-sharing in the Haight: some social and psychological functions', *Journal of Health and Social Behaviour*, 11: 220–230.

Humphreys, L. (1970) *Tearoom Trade: Impersonal Sex in Public Places*. Chicago: Aldine.

Hunt, A., Christofinis, G., Coxon, A. et al. (1990) 'Seroprevalence of HIV-1 infection in a cohort of homosexually active men', *Genitourinary Medicine*, 66: 423–427.

Hunt, A., Davies, P., Weatherburn, P. et al. (1991) 'Changes in sexual behaviour in a large cohort of homosexual men in England and Wales, 1988–9', *British Medical Journal*, 302: 505–506.

Hunt, A., Davies, P., McManus, T., et al. (1992) 'HIV-1 infection in a cohort of gay and bisexual men', *British Medical Journal*, 305: 561–562.

Ikonga, M., Boupda, A., Betima, J. et al. (1992) 'Peer educators as condom distributors among high risk groups in Yaounde, Cameroon'. Paper presented at VIII International Conference on AIDS, Amsterdam [abstract PoD 5635].

Izazola, J., Gortmaker, S., Basanez, R. and Sepulveda, J. (1991) 'Sexual relationships with women in homosexually identified men'. Paper presented at VII International Conference on AIDS, Florence [abstract M.C. 102].

Jay, P., Stall, R., Crosby, M. et al. (1992) 'Understanding high-risk sexual behaviour among gay male substance abusers'. Paper presented at VIII International Conference on AIDS, Amsterdam [abstract PoD 5193].

Johnson, A. (1988) 'Heterosexual transmission of human immunodeficiency virus', *British Medical Journal*, 296: 1017–1020.

Johnson, A. and Gill, N. (1989) 'Evidence for recent changes in sexual behaviour in homosexual men in England and Wales', *Philosophical Transactions Royal Society London*, B325: 153–161.

Johnson, A. and Laga, M. (1990) 'Heterosexual transmission of HIV', in N. Alexander, H. Gabelnick and J. Spieler (eds) *Heterosexual Transmission of AIDS*. New York: Wiley-Liss, pp. 9–22.

Johnson, A., Wadsworth, J., Field, J. et al. (1990) 'Surveying sexual lifestyles', *Nature*, 343: 109.

Johnson, A., Wadsworth, J., Wellings, K. et al. (1992) 'Sexual lifestyles and HIV risk', *Nature*, 360: 410–412.

Johnson, A., Wadsworth, J., Wellings, K. and Field, J. (1994) *Sexual Attitudes and Lifestyles*. Oxford: Blackwell.

Johnson, B. (1987) 'The environmentalist movement and grid/group analysis: a modest critique', in B. Johnson and V. Corvello (eds) *The Social and Cultural Construction of Risk*. Dordrecht: Reidel.

Joseph, J., Montgomery, S., Emmons, C. et al. (1987) 'Perceived risk of AIDS: assessing the behavioural and psychosocial consequences in a cohort of gay men', *Journal of Applied Social Psychology*, 17: 231–250.

Kaslow, R. et al. (1987) 'Multicenter AIDS cohort study: rationale, organization and selected characteristics of the participants', *American Journal of Epidemiology*, 126: 310–318.

Kaye, P. and Miller, E. (1991) 'Incidence of HIV-1 infection in an opportunistic cohort of male homosexuals in England during 1986-90'. Paper presented at VII International Conference on AIDS, Florence [abstract W.C. 3000].

Kefenie, H., Desta, B., Zewdie, D. (1992) 'HIV-1 Seroprevalence in Ethiopia – 5 years interval'. Paper presented at VIII International Conference on AIDS, Amsterdam [abstract PoC 4017].

Kelly, J., Lawrence, J., Hood, H. and Brasfield, T. (1989) 'Behavioural intervention to reduce AIDS risk activities', *Journal of Clinical and Consulting Psychology*, 57: 60–67.

Kelly, J. Lawrence, J., Diaz, Y. et al. (1991) 'HIV risk reduction following intervention with key opinion leaders of population: an experimental analysis', *American Journal of Public Health*, 81: 168–171.

Kelly, J., Sikkema, K., Winett, R. et al. (1992) 'Outcomes of a sixteen city randomised field trial of a community-level HIV risk reduction intervention'. Paper presented at VIII International Conference on AIDS, Amsterdam, 1992 [abstract TuD 0543].

Kent, V., Davies, M., Deverell, K. and Gottesman, S. (1990) 'Social interaction routines involved in heterosexual encounters: prelude to first intercourse'. Paper presented at Fourth Conference on Social Aspects of AIDS. London: South Bank Polytechnic.

Keogh, P., Church, J., Vearnals, S. and Green, J. (1992) 'Investigation of motivational and behavioural factors influencing men who have sex with men in public toilets (cottaging)'. Paper presented at VIII International Conference on AIDS, Amsterdam [abstract PoD 5187].

Killinger, J., Kroner, N., White, G. et al. (1990) 'Safe sex practices of female partners of haemophiliac men'. Paper presented at VI International Conference on AIDS, San Francisco [abstract 3019].

Kingsley, L. et al. (1991) 'Temporal trends in human immunodeficiency virus type 1. Seroconversion 1984–1989', *American Journal of Epidemiology*, 134: 331–339.

Kinsey, A., Pomeroy, W. and Martin, C. (1948) *Sexual Behaviour in the Human Male*. Philadelphia: W.B. Saunders.

Kinsey, A., Pomeroy, W., Martin, C. and Gebhard, P. (1953) *Sexual Behaviour in the Human Female*. Philadelphia: W.B. Saunders.

Kippax, S., Connell, R., Dowsett, G. and Crawford, J. (1993) *Sustaining Safe Sex*. London: Falmer.

Kitzinger, J. and Miller, D. (1992) 'African AIDS: audience understandings of media messages', in P. Aggleton et al. (eds) *AIDS: Rights, Risk and Reason*. London: Falmer.

Klee, H., Faugier, J., Hayes, C. et al. (1990a) 'AIDS-related risk behaviour, poly-drug use and Temazepam', *British Journal of Addiction*, 85: 1125–1132.

Klee, H., Faugier, J., Hayes, C. et al. (1990b) 'Factors associated with risk behaviour among injecting drug users', *AIDS Care*, 2: 133–145.

Kleiber, D., Wilke, M. and Kreilkamp, E. (1991) 'Aids and sex tourism'. Paper presented at VII International Conference on AIDS, Florence [abstract M.D. 4037].

Korkia, P. and Stimson, G. (1993) *Anabolic Steroid Use in Great Britain. Report to the Departments of Health of England, Scotland and Wales*. London: Centre for Research on Drugs and Health Behaviour.

Kronenfeld, J. (1988) 'Models of preventive health behaviour, health behaviour change, and roles for sociologists', *Research in the Sociology of Health Care*, 7: 303–328.

Kronenfeld, J. and Glik, D. (1991) 'Perceptions of risk: its applicability in medical sociological research', *Research in the Sociology of Health Care*, 9: 307–334.

Kunanusont, C., Weniger, B., Foy, H. et al. (1991) 'Modes of transmission for the high rates of HIV infection among male STD patients and male blood donors in Chianymai, Thailand'. Paper presented at VII International Conference on AIDS, Florence [abstract W.C. 3086].

Laga, M., Nzila, N. and Goeman, J. (1991) 'The inter-relationship of sexually transmitted diseases and HIV infection: implications for the control of both epidemics in Africa', *AIDS 5* (suppl. 1): S55–S63.

Lampinen, T., Joo, E., Seweryn, S. et al. (1992) 'HIV seropositivity in community-recruited and drug treatment samples of injecting drug users', *AIDS*, 6: 123–126.

Landis, S., Schoenbach, V., Weber, D. et al. (1992) 'Results of a randomized trial of partner notification in cases of HIV infection in North Carolina', *New England Journal of Medicine*, 326: 101–106.

Larson, A. (1989) 'Social context of Human Immunodeficiency Virus transmission in Africa: historical and cultural bases of East and Central African sexual relations', *Reviews of Infectious Diseases*, 11: 716–731.

Leigh Brown, A. (1992) 'The biology of HIV transmission'. Paper presented at MRC AIDS Epidemiology Workshop, Heriot-Watt University, Edinburgh.

Louie, L., Just, J., Padian, N. and King, M. (1991) 'Genetic marker for susceptibility to heterosexual HIV-1 infection'. Paper presented at VII International Conference on AIDS, Florence [abstract M.C. 3091].

Louis, F., Garcia-Calleja, J., Zekeng, L. et al. (1993) 'HIV seroprevalence among Bantous and Pygmies in South Cameroon: a comparative study at a four year interval (1990–1993)'. Paper presented at IX International Conference on AIDS, Berlin [abstract PO–CO7–2754].

Luker, K. (1975) *Taking Chances: Abortion and the Decision not to Contracept*. Berkeley: University of California Press.

Maardh, P. and Kallings, I. (1990) 'Tourism has a great impact on the epidemiology of sexually transmitted diseases: emphasis on a European perspective', in W. Pasini (ed.) *Tourist Health*. Rimini: WHO Collaborating Centre for Tourist Health and Medicine. Cited in Hendriks (1991).

Macintyre, S. and West, P. (1993) '"What does the phrase safer sex mean to you?" Understandings among Glaswegian 18 year olds in 1990', *AIDS*, 7: 121–125.

McKeganey, N. (1990) 'Being positive: drug injectors' experiences of HIV infection', *British Journal of Addiction*, 85: 1113–1124.

McKeganey, N. (1994) 'Prostitution and HIV: what do we know and where might research be targeted in future?', *AIDS*, 8: 1215–1226.

McKeganey, M. and Barnard, M. (1992) *AIDS, Drugs and Sexual Risk: Lives in the Balance*. Buckingham: Open University Press.

McKeganey, N., Barnard, M. and Bloor, M. (1990) 'A comparison of HIV related risk behaviour and risk reduction between female streetworking prostitutes and rent boys in Glasgow', *Sociology of Health and Illness*, 12: 274–292.

McKeganey, N., Barnard, M., Leyland, A. et al. (1992) 'Female prostitution and HIV infection in Glasgow', *British Medical Journal*, 305: 801–804.

Mackworth, J. (1969) *Vigilance and Habituation*. Harmondsworth: Penguin.

Macmillan, J. (1975) *Deviant Drivers*. Farnborough: Saxon House.

McMullen, R. (1990) *Male Rape: Breaking the Silence on the Last Taboo*. London: GMP.

Mamor, M., Des Jarlais, D., Cohen, H. et al. (1987) 'Risk factors for infection with HIV among intravenous drug abusers in New York City', *AIDS*, 1: 39–44.

Mann, J.M. (1991) 'Global AIDS: critical issues for prevention in the 1990s', *International Journal of Health Services*, 21: 553–559.

M'Boup, S., Kauki, P., N'Doye, I. et al. (1990) 'Emergence of HIV-1 in a high risk group from an HIV-2 endemic area (Senegal)'. Paper presented at VI International Conference on AIDS, San Francisco [abstract F.C. 1023].

Mechanic, D. (1962) 'The concept of illness behaviour', *Journal of Chronic Diseases*, 15: 189–194.

Moodie, D. (with Ndatsche, V. and Sibuyi, B.) (1988) 'Migrancy and male sexuality in the South African gold mines', *Journal of Southern African Studies*, 14: 228–256.

Morin, E. (1971) *Rumour in Orleans*. London: Antony Blond.

Morse, E., Simon, P., Osofsky, H. et al. (1991) 'The male street prostitute: a vector for the transmission of HIV infection into the heterosexual world', *Social Science and Medicine*, 32: 535–539.

Moses, S., Plummer, E.A., Ngugi, E.N. et al. (1991) 'Controlling HIV in Africa: effectiveness and cost of an intervention in a high frequency STD transmitter core group', *AIDS*, 5: 407–411.

Moss, A. (1987) 'AIDS and intravenous drug use: the real heterosexual epidemic', *British Medical Journal*, 294: 389–390.

Moss, A. (1988) 'Epidemiology of AIDS in developed countries', *British Medical Bulletin*, 44: 56–67.

Monzon, O.T., Santana, R.T., Paladin, F.J.E. et al. (1990) 'Condom use and sexually transmitted diseases among commercial sex workers undergoing a health education/intervention programme on AIDS in the Philippines'. Paper presented at VI International Conference on AIDS, San Francisco [abstract Th.D. 778].

Mulder, D.W., Kengeya-Kayonda, J.F. and Sempala, S.D.K. (1991) 'MRC (UK) programme on AIDS in Uganda'. Paper presented at MRC AIDS Epidemiology Warwick Workshop.

Naik, T.N., Sarkar, S., Singh, H.C., Bhunia, S.C. et al. (1991) 'Intravenous drug users – a new high-risk group for HIV infection in India', *AIDS*, 5: 117–118.

Noone, A., MacDonald, N., Evans, B. and Heptonstall, J. (1992) 'HIV transmission, travel and Thailand' (letter), *Lancet*, 305: 892.

Nyirenda-Meya, J. (1992) 'A study of the behavioural aspects of dry sex practice in Lusaka'. Paper presented at VIII International Conference on AIDS, Amsterdam [abstract PoD 5448].

Nzila, N., Luga, M., Thiam, M. et al. (1991) 'HIV and other sexually transmitted diseases among female prostitutes in Kinshasa', *AIDS*, 5: 715–721.

Padian, N. (1990) 'Heterosexual transmission: infectivity and risks', in N. Alexander, H. Gabelnick and J. Spieler (eds) *Heterosexual Transmission of AIDS*. New York: Wiley-Liss, pp. 25–33.

Padian, N., Marquis, L., Francis, D. et al. (1987) 'Male to female transmission of human immunodeficiency virus', *Journal of American Medical Association*, 258: 788–790.

Palacio, V., Vazquez, S., Quiros, R. et al. (1989) 'Incidence of HIV in prostitutes in Oviedo, Spain', *AIDS*, 3: 461–463.

Panos Institute (1989) *AIDS and the Third World*. Philadelphia: New Society.

Parker, H., Bax, K. and Newcombe, R. (1988) *Living with Heroin*. Buckingham: Open University Press.

Parker, R. (1987) 'Acquired Immune Deficiency Syndrome in urban Brazil', *Medical Anthropology Quarterly* 1: 155–175.

Parkin, D. (1978) *The Cultural Definition of Political Response*. London: Academic Press.

Parsons, E. (1990) 'Living with Duchene Muscular Dystrophy: women's understandings of disability and risk'. PhD thesis, University of Wales College of Cardiff.

Parsons, E. and Atkinson, P. (1992) 'Lay constructions of genetic risk', *Sociology of Health and Illness*, 14: 437–455.

Pates, R. and Temple, D. (1992) *The Use of Anabolic Steroids in Wales*. Cardiff: Welsh Committee on Drug Misuse.

Patton, C. (1985) *Sex and Germs: the Politics of AIDS*. Boston: Southend Press.

Pattullo, A., Plourde, P., Ndinya-Achola, J. et al. (1992) 'Prospective study of HIV-1 seroconversion in women with genital ulcers attending an African STD clinic'. Paper presented at VIII International Conference on AIDS, Amsterdam [abstract PoC 4326].

Pavia, A., Benyo, M., Niler, L. and Risk, H. (1993) 'Partner notification for control of HIV: results after 2 years of a statewide program in Utah', *American Journal of Public Health*, 83: 1418–1424.

Peckham, C. (1993) Paper presented to MRC AIDS Programme Workshop, University of Sussex, Brighton.

Pepin, J., Dunn, D., Gage, I. et al. (1991) 'HIV-2 infection among prostitutes working in the Gambia: association with serological evidence of genital ulcer diseases and with generalised lymphadenopathy', *AIDS*, 5: 1127–1132.

Perlongher, N. (1987) 'Vicissitudes des garçons de la nuit', *Revisto Temes do IMESC* (São Paulo), 4: 1–21.

PHLS Working Group (1993) 'The incidence and prevalence of AIDS and other severe HIV diseases in England and Wales for 1992–1997: projections using data to the end of June 1992 (revised Day Report)', *Communicable Disease Report*, 3, suppl. 1.

Phongpaichit, P. (1982) *From Peasant Girls to Bangkok Masseuses*. Geneva: International Labor Organization.

Pickering, H., Todd, J., Dunn, D. et al. (1992) 'Prostitutes and their clients: a Gambian survey', *Social Science and Medicine*, 34: 75–88.

Plant, M. (1990) 'Alcohol, sex and AIDS', *Alcohol and Alcoholism*, 25: 293–301.

Plummer, F.A., Nagelkerke, N.J.D., Moses, S. et al. (1991) 'The importance of core groups in the epidemiology and control of HIV-1 infection', *AIDS*, 5 (suppl. 1): S169–S176.

Pokrovsky, V., Eramova, I., Savchenko, I. et al. (1991) 'HIV transmission in the USSR'. Paper presented at VII International Conference on AIDS, Florence [abstract W.C. 3056].

Prout, A. and Deverell, K. (1994) *MESMAC Working with Diversity – building Communities: an Evaluation of a Community Development Approach to HIV Prevention for Men who have Sex with Men*. London: Health Education Authority.

Public Health Laboratory Service (1991) 'The unlinked anonymous HIV prevalence programme in England and Wales: preliminary results', *Communicable Disease Report*, 1, review 7: R69–R76.

Public Health Laboratory Service (1994) *Communicable Disease Report*, 4.

Quinn, T.C. et al. (1986) 'AIDS in Africa – an epidemiological paradigm', *Science*, 234: 935–963.

Rainwater, L. (1968) 'The lower class: health, illness and medical institutions', in I. Deutscher and E. Thompson (eds) *Among the People*. New York: Basic Books.

Rayner, S. (1986) 'Management of radiation hazards in hospitals: plural rationalities in a single institution', *Social Studies of Science*, 16: 573–591.

Reardon, J., Gaudino, J., Wilson, M. et al. (1991) 'Epidemiology of HIV-1 in intravenous drug users in treatment in the San Francisco Bay area, California, 1989–1990'. Paper presented at VII International Conference on AIDS, Florence [abstract M.C. 3221].

Reckhart, M., Manzon, L. and Tucker, P. (1993) 'Transexuals and AIDS'. Paper presented at IX International Conference on AIDS, Berlin [abstract PO–C21–3101].

Rhodes, T. and Stimson, G. (forthcoming) 'Sex, drugs, intervention and research: from the individual to the social', *International Journal of the Addictions*.

Rhodes, T., Hartnoll, R., Johnson, A. et al. (1991) *Out of the Agency and on to the Streets: a Review of HIV Outreach Health Education in Europe and the United States*. ISSD Research Monograph 2. London: Institute for the Study of Drug Dependence.

Rhodes, T., Bloor, M., Donoghoe, M. et al. (1993) 'HIV prevalence and HIV risk behaviour among injecting drug users in London and Glasgow', *AIDS Care*, 5: 4413–4425.

Ricard, D., Wilkins, A., N'Gum, P. et al (1994) 'The effects of HIV-2 infection in a rural area of Guinea-Bissau', *AIDS*, 8: 977–982.

Riley, V. (1991) 'Resurgent gonorrhoea in homosexual men', *Lancet*, 1: 183.

Robertson, C. (1984) 'Women in the urban economy', in M. Hays and S. Stichter (eds) *African Women South of the Sahara*. London: Longmans.

Robertson, R., Bucknall, A., Welsby, P. et al. (1986) 'Epidemic of AIDS-related virus infection among intravenous drug users', *British Medical Journal*, 292: 527–529.

Ronald, P., Robertson, R. and Roberts, J. (1992) 'Risk-taking behaviour on the decline in intravenous drug users', *British Journal of Addiction*, 87: 115–116.

Rosenstock, I. (1966) 'Why people use health services', *Millbank Memorial Fund Quarterly*, 44: 94–124.

Rosenstock, I. (1974) 'The health belief model and preventive health behaviour', *Health Education Monographs*, 2: 354–386.

Royal Society (1992) *Risk Analysis, Perception and Management: Report of a Royal Society Study Group*. London: Royal Society.

Sato, P.A., Chin, J. and Mann, J.M. (1989) 'Review of AIDS and HIV prevention: global epidemiology and statistics', *AIDS*, 3 (suppl.): S301–307.

Schrott-Ben Redjeb, G., Pant, A. and Kleiber, D. (1992) 'Sexual conduct and sexual identity in clients of male sexworkers'. Paper presented at VIII International Conference on AIDS, Amsterdam [abstract PoD 5656].

Schutz, A. (1970) *Reflections on the Problem of Relevance*. New Haven: Yale University Press.

Schutz, A. and Luckmann, T. (1974) *The Structure of the Social World*. London: Heinemann.

Scott, M. and Lyman, B. (1968) 'Accounts', *American Sociological Review*, 33: 46–63.

Seibt, A., Ross, M., Freeman, A. et al. (1994) 'Relationship between safe sex and acculturation into the gay community'. Paper presented at Second International Conference on Biopsychosocial Aspects of HIV Infection, Brighton [abstract PO 37].

Shannuganaudan, S., Uma, A. and Thirumalaikolundusubramanian, P. (1994) 'Socioeconomic impact of AIDS: identification of major dimensions and planning for health care in India'. Paper presented at Second International Conference on Biopsychosocial Aspects of HIV Infection, Brighton [abstract PO 130].

Shilts, R. (1987) *And the Band Played On: People, Politics and the AIDS Crisis*. London: Penguin.

Siegal, H., Baumgartner, K., Carlson, R. et al. (1991) 'HIV infection and risk behaviours among injectable drug users in low seroprevalence areas in the Midwest'. Paper presented at VII International Conference on AIDS, Florence [abstract M.C. 3213].

Sittitrai, W., Wongsukoi, N., Phanuphak, P. and Brown, T. (1993) 'Female commercial sex workers in Thailand – prevalence and risk determinants'. Paper presented at IX International Conference on AIDS, Berlin [abstract PO–D09–3653].

Skegg, D. (1989) 'Heterosexually acquired HIV infection: still hard to be sure about a future epidemic', *British Medical Journal*, 298: 401–402.

Sorensen, J., Giydish, J., Constantini, M. and Balstic, S. (1989) 'Changes in needle-sharing and syringe-cleaning among San Francisco drug abusers', *New England Journal of Medicine*, 320: 807.

Soro, B., Moreau, J., Gershy-Danet, G. et al. (1990) 'Progression of the epidemic in West Africa'. Paper presented at VI International Conference on AIDS, San Francisco [abstract Th.C. 719]

Stall, R., Ekstrand, M., Pollack, L. et al. (1990) 'Relapse from safer sex: the next challenge for AIDS prevention efforts', *Journal of the Acquired Immune Deficiency Syndromes*, 3: 1181–1187.

Stevens, C., Taylor, P., Zang, E. et al. (1986) 'Human T-cell lymphotrophic virus type III infection in a cohort of homosexual men in New York City', *Journal of American Medical Association*, 255: 2167–2172.

Stigum, H., Grennesby, J., Magnus, P. et al. (1989) 'The potential for spread of HIV in the heterosexual population in Norway, a simulation model study'. Paper presented at V International Conference on AIDS, Montreal [abstract Th.A.P. 59].

Stimson, G. (1993) 'The global diffusion of injecting drug use: implications for HIV infection', *Bulletin of Narcotics*, 45: 3–17.

Stimson, G. (1994a) 'AIDS and drug use – five years on', Third Dorothy Black Lecture, Charing Cross and Westminster Medical School, London.

Stimson, G. (1994b) 'The role of drug-injecting in the spread of HIV infection in South East Asia'. Plenary paper, Second International Conference on Biopsychosocial Aspects of HIV infection, Brighton.

Stimson, G. (forthcoming) 'AIDS and injecting drug use in the United Kingdom, 1988 to 1993: the policy response and the prevention of the epidemic', *Social Science and Medicine*.

Stimson, G. and Oppenheimer, E. (1982) *Heroin Addiction: treating and control*. London: Tavistock.

Stimson, G., Alldritt, L., Dolan, K. and Donoghoe, M. (1988a) 'Syringe-exchange schemes for drug users in England and Scotland', *British Medical Journal*, 296: 1717–1719.

Stimson, G., Alldrit, L., Donoghoe, M. and Lart, R. (1988b) *Injecting Equipment Exchange Schemes: Final Report*. London: Goldsmiths College.

Stimson, G., Keene, J., Parry-Langdon, N. and Jones, S. (1992) *Evaluation of the Syringe-Exchange Programme in Wales. Final Report to the Welsh Office*. London: Centre for Research on Drugs and Health Behaviour.

Stoneburner, R., Chiasson, M., Weisfuse, I. and Thomas, P. (1990) 'The epidemic of AIDS and HIV-1 infection among heterosexuals in New York City', *AIDS*, 4: 99–106.

Strauss, A. (1969) 'Medical organisation, medical care, and lower income groups', *Social Science and Medicine*, 3: 143–177.

Studemeister, A., Westling, R. and Kent, G. (1990) 'HIV infection among immigrants to the United States'. Paper presented at VI International Conference on AIDS, San Francisco [abstract FC 547].

Suchman, E. (1965) 'Socio-medical variations among ethnic groups', *American Journal of Sociology*, 70: 319–331.

Sugarman, B. (1974) *Daytop Village – a Therapeutic Community*. New York: Holt, Rinehart and Winston.

Sundet, J., Kvalem, I., Magnus, P. and Bakketeig, L. (1988) 'Prevalence of risk-prone sexual behaviour in the general population of Norway', in A. Fleming et al. (eds) *Global Impact of AIDS*. New York: Alan Liss, pp. 53–60.

Tabet, S., Palmer, D., Voorhees, R. and Wiese, W. (1991) 'Prostitutes, drug use and HIV/AIDS on the streets of Albuquerque, New Mexico'. Paper presented at VII International Conference on AIDS, Florence [abstract M.C. 3216].

Taylor, A., Frischer, M., Green, S. et al. (1994) 'Low and stable prevalence of HIV among Glasgow drug injectors', *International Journal of STD and AIDS*, 5: 105–107.

Telzak, E., Chiasson, M., Bevier, P. et al. (1991) 'Chancroid and the high risk of HIV seroconversion in male heterosexuals in New York City'. Paper presented at VII International Conference on AIDS, Florence [abstract W.C. 45].

Tempesta, E. and Di Giannantonio, M. (1990) 'The Italian epidemic: a case study', in J. Strang and G. Stimson (eds) *AIDS and Drug Misuse*. London: Routledge, pp. 63–74.

Thomas, W.I. (1964) 'The definition of the situation', in L. Coser and B. Rosenberg (eds) *Sociological Theory: a Book of Readings*. New York: Collier-Macmillan.

Tirelli, U., Rezza, G., Ginliani, M. et al. (1989) 'HIV seroprevalence among 304 female prostitutes from four Italian towns' (letter), *AIDS*, 3: 547–548.

Tokars, J., Marcus, R., Culver, D. et al. (1990) 'Zidovudine (AZT) use after occupational exposure to HIV-infected blood'. Paper presented at VI International Conference on AIDS, San Francisco [abstract S.C. 766].

Tomlinson, D. et al. (1991a) 'Does rectal gonorrhoea reflect unsafe sex?', *Lancet*, 1: 501–502.

Tomlinson, D., Hillman, R., Harris, J. and Taylor-Robinson, D. (1991b) 'Screening for sexually transmitted disease in London-based male prostitutes', *Genitourinary Medicine*, 67: 103–106.

Treichler, P. (1992) 'AIDS, HIV and the cultural construction of reality', in G. Herdt and S. Lindenbaum (eds) *The Time of AIDS*. Newbury Park: Sage.

Tuliza, M., Manoka, A., Nzila, N. et al. (1991) 'The impact of STD control and condom promotion on the incidence of HIV in Kinshasa prostitutes'. Paper presented at VII International Conference on AIDS, Florence [abstract M.C. 2].

Turnbull, P., Dolan, K. and Stimson, G. (1990) 'HIV-related risk behaviour among prisoners', *British Medical Journal*, 85: 123–135.

Turner, C. (1989) 'Research on sexual behaviours that transmit HIV: progress and problems', *AIDS*, 3 (suppl. 1): S63–S69.

Ungchusak, K., Thanprasertsuk, S., Sriprapandh, S. et al. (1990) 'First national sentinel seroprevalence survey for HIV-1 infection in Thailand, June 1989'. Paper presented at VI International Conference on AIDS, San Francisco [abstract F.C. 99].

Van Buuren, N.G. and Longo, P.H. (1991) 'New strategies to prevent HIV infection among the partners/lovers of street boys involved in prostitution'. Paper presented at VII International Conference on AIDS, Florence [abstract W.C. 3029].

Van den Hoek, J. et al. (1990) 'Increase in unsafe homosexual behaviour', *Lancet*, 2: 179–180.

Van Griensven, G., de Vroome, E., Goudsmit, J. and Coutinho, R. (1989) 'Changes in sexual behaviour and the fall in the incidence of HIV infection among homosexual men', *British Medical Journal*, 298: 218–221.

Van Haastrecht, H., van den Hoek, J., Mientjes, G. and Coutinho, R. (1991) 'Did the introduction of HIV among homosexual men precede the introduction of HIV among injecting drug users in the Netherlands?' (letter) *AIDS*, 6: 131–132.

Vanichseni, S., Sonchai, W., Plangsringarm, K. et al. (1989) 'Second seroprevalence survey among Bangkok's intravenous drug addicts'. Paper presented at V International Conference on AIDS, Montreal [abstract T.G.O. 23].

Vorakitphokatorn, S. and Cash, R. (1992) 'Factors that determine condom use among traditionally high users: Japanese men and commercial sex workers in Bangkok, Thailand'. Paper presented at VIII International Conference on AIDS, Amsterdam [abstract PoD 5239].

Vuksanovic, P. and Low, A. (1991) 'Venereal diseases and AIDS among seafarers', *Travel Medicine*, 9: 121–123.

Watney, S. (1987) *Policing Desire: Pornography, AIDS and the Media*. London: Comedia.

Weatherburn, P., Davies, P., Hunt, A. et al. (1992) 'Heterosexual behaviour in a large cohort of homosexually active men in England and Wales', *AIDS Care*, 2: 319–324.

Weatherburn, P., Stephens, M., Reid, D. et al. (1994) 'Age does not predict unprotected anal intercourse'. Paper presented at Second International Conference on Biopsychosocial Aspects of HIV Infection, Brighton [abstract PO 25].

Weinstein, N. (1988) 'The precaution adoption process', *Health Psychology*, 7: 355–386.

Weiss, S., Ginzburg, H., Goedert, J. et al. (1985) 'Risk for HTLV-III exposure and AIDS among parenteral drug abusers in New Jersey'. Paper presented at First International Conference on AIDS, Atlanta.

Wellings, K. (1992) 'EC concerted action: assessment of the AIDS/HIV prevention strategies in the general population'. Paper presented at VIII International Conference on AIDS, Amsterdam [abstract PoD 5346].

Wellings, K., Field, J., Johnson, A. and Wadsworth, J. (1994) *Sexual Behaviour in Britain*. Harmondsworth: Penguin.

WHO Collaborative Study Group (1993) 'An international comparative study of HIV prevalence and risk behaviour among drug injectors in 13 cities', *Bulletin of Narcotics*, 45: 19–45.

Wight, D. (1993) 'Constraint or cognition? Factors affecting young men's practice of safer heterosexual sex', in P. Aggleton, P. Davies and G. Hart (eds) *AIDS: The Second Decade*. Lewes: Falmer.

Wight, D. (1994) 'The diversity of working class men's heterosexual relationships at 19 years'. Paper presented at British Sociological Association Annual Conference, Preston.

Wilke, M. and Kleiber, D. (1991) 'AIDS and sex tourism'. Paper presented at VII International Conference on AIDS, Florence [abstract M.D. 4037].

Wilke, M. and Kleiber, D. (1992) 'Sexual behaviour of gay German tourists in Thailand'. Paper presented at VIII International Conference on AIDS, Amsterdam [abstract PoD 5239].

Wilkins, A., Hayes, R., Alonso, P. et al. (1991) 'Risk factors for HIV-2 infection in the Gambia', *AIDS*, 5: 1127–1132.

Wilkins, A., Ricard, D., Todd, J. et al. (1993) 'The epidemiology of HIV infection in a rural area of Guinea-Bissau', *AIDS*, 7: 1119–1122.

Wilson, D., Mavasere, D. and Katuria, R. (1991) 'Ethnographic and quantitative research to design a community-based intervention among commercial fishermen on Lake Kariba, Zimbabwe'. Paper presented at VII International Conference on AIDS, Florence [abstract W.D. 4042].

Winkelstein, W., Wiley, J., Padian, N. et al. (1988) 'The San Francisco Men's Health Study: continued decline in HIV seroconversion rates among homosexual/bisexual men', *American Journal of Public Health*, 78: 1472–1474.

Wirawan, D., Fajans, P. and Ford, K. (1992) 'Sexual behaviour and condom use among male sex workers and male tourist clients in Bali, Indonesia'. Paper presented at VIII International Conference on AIDS, Amsterdam [abstract PoD 5240].

Wong, M., Tan, M., Ho, J. et al. (1994) 'Knowledge and sexual behaviour related to HIV and AIDS of female sex workers in Singapore', *Health Education Journal*, 53: 155–162.

Yorke, J.A., Hethcote, H.W. and Nold, A. (1978) 'Dynamics and control of the transmission of gonorrhoea', *Sexually Transmitted Diseases*, 5: 31–36.

Zheng, X., Tian, C., Choi, K-H. et al. (1994) 'Injecting drug use and HIV infection in S.W. China', *AIDS*, 8: 1141–1147.

Zola, I. (1973) 'Pathways to the doctor: from person to patient', *Social Science and Medicine*, 7: 677–689.

Index